Intermittent Fasting 16/8

The 16/8 method as the best option to lose weight, regenerate your body, increase your energy, control your hunger and feel better. A step-by-step guide to change your image and your lifestyle

Paty Breads

© Copyright 2019 by Paty Breads - All rights reserved.

This Book is provided with the sole purpose of providing relevant information on a specific topic for which every reasonable effort has been made to ensure that it is both accurate and reasonable. Nevertheless, by purchasing this Book you consent to the fact that the author, as well as the publisher, are in no way experts on the topics contained herein, regardless of any claims as such that may be made within. As such, any suggestions or recommendations that are made within are done so purely for entertainment value. It is recommended that you always consult a professional prior to undertaking any of the advice or techniques discussed within.

This is a legally binding declaration that is considered both valid and fair by both the Committee of Publishers Association and the American Bar Association and should be considered as legally binding within the United States.

The reproduction, transmission, and duplication of any of the content found herein, including any specific or extended information will be done as an illegal act regardless of the end form the information ultimately takes. This includes copied versions of the work, both physical, digital, and audio, unless the express consent of the Publisher is provided beforehand. Any additional rights reserved.

Furthermore, the information that can be found within the pages described forthwith shall be considered both accurate and truthful when it comes to the recounting of facts. As such, any use, correct or incorrect, of the provided information will render the Publisher free of responsibility as to the actions taken outside of their direct purview. Regardless, there are zero scenarios where the original author or the Publisher can be deemed liable in any fashion for any damages or hardships that may result from any of the information discussed herein.

Additionally, the information in the following pages is intended only for informational purposes and should thus be thought of as universal. As befitting its nature, it is presented without assurance regarding its prolonged validity or interim quality. Trademarks that are mentioned are done without written consent and can in no way be considered an endorsement from the trademark holder.

Table of Contents

Introduction

Chapter 1: The Problem with Modern Diet

    What Are Issues with Modern Diet?

    Avoid Unhealthy Eating Habits

    Listen to Your Body

    No One Is Perfect

    How to Change Bad Habits

    Brush Your Teeth After Dinner to Reduce the Temptation to Eat.

Chapter 2: Intermitted Fasting, What Is It?

    Intermittent Fasting History

    Fasting Science

    Circadian Rhythm Biology

    This Is a Place for Temporary Fasting.

    Microbiome of the Gut Microbiome

        Slow down

        Life Behavior

    Why Do You Want to Fast?

    Intermittent Fasting Types

Chapter 3: How Do You Fast?

  The 16:8 Method

    16:8 Schedule

  Factors to Consider for Achieving Success

    Goal Setting

  Collection

  Support

  Maintain Discipline

  Patience Pays

  Have a Clear Mind

  Effective Reliability

  Confidence

  Resetting

  Productivity

  Rest

  Tips to Help You Sleep Well

    Get Enough Sunlight

    Avoid Watching Before You Go to Bed

    Dark Sleep

    Quality Is Not Quantity

    Power

Stay Strong

Try to Avoid Your Temptation.

Prepare Your Refrigerator to Make Fasting Days Easier.

Remember That Social Meeting Does Not Have to Be Included in Food.

If You Are a Sanitizer, Stay Away from the Triggers.

Reward Yourself

Learn to Tell the Difference Between Hunger and Other Emotions.

Other Ways of Intermittent Fasting

Diet 5:2

Eat a Regular Diet

Another Fasting Day

Worrier Food

Skipping Meals Spontaneously

Chapter 4: Why Should You Do Intermittent Fasting?

It Modulates the Cells, Hormones and Genes Function

Weight Loss and Body Fat

It Helps with Diabetes

Simplifying Life

Good on the Heart

Can Help with Cancer

Good on the Mind

It Helps to Improve Cells

May Prevent Alzheimer's Disease

Regular Fasting Can Help You Live Longer

Issues Associated with Being Overweight

Diseases of Behavior

Osteoarthritis

Sleep Apnea

Stroke

Understanding Your Body and Intermittent Fasting

Cleaning System

The Journey to Having a Successful Fasting Program Can Be Very Difficult.

Chapter 5: Successful, Fasting, Eating and Eating

Exercise While Maintaining Muscle Mass

Exercise and Fasting Together

Use Your Fitness Tips a Lot

Reduce the Number of Times and Gain Weight Is Best for Soft Muscles - If at All

Chapter 6: Intermittent Fasting Diet.

How This Fat Is Stored and Burnt?

How Is Energy Stored in Our Bodies?

How Is the Stored Energy Used in Body Functioning?

Hormones

Human Growth Hormone (HGM)

Leptin

Using the Ketogenic Diet with Intermittent Fasting

Chapter 7: Tips to Help You Succeed in Intermittent Fasting

Ride out the Hunger Waves

Start Gradually

Chapter 8: Most FAQ(s) on Intermitted Fasting

Who Should Fast and Not?

Can Someone Starve While Fasting?

What Side Effects Do They Come with Fasting?

How to Manage the Hunger

Can Fasting Burn Muscle?

Can Women Fast?

Bonus Tips to Help in Maintaining the Proper Weight

Use of Spices

Cinnamon

Ginger

Onion and Garlic

Turmeric

Cayenne Pepper

Black Pepper

Cumin

Tea of Different Flavors

Herbal Water

Reduce Salt and Sugar Intake

Rules to Consider

Invalid Weight Loss Method

Fat-Free and Sugar-Free

Loading Protein

Counting Calories

Keep Away from Snacks

Low-Calorie Diet

Get Rid of Dairy Products

Detoxification

Skip Breakfast

Fast Food

Go out for Meal

Learn How Japanese Maintain Their Weight

Avoid Milk

Optimize Food Temperature

Healthy Snack

Not Every Night Is a Sweet Night

Rice Combination

Seafood

Small Plates and Chopsticks

3:1 Rationing

Soup Plan

Extreme Drink

Conclusion

Introduction

Fasting doesn't mean not eating; it's about eating with planning. It's a way to plan your meals so you can benefit more. Intermittent fasting involves changing the way you eat but not the kinds of foods you eat.

Well, in particular, it's the best way to treat it without eating crazy foods or lowering your calories for nothing. Most times you will try to keep your calories the same when you start a non-stop fast. (Most people eat large meals over a short period.) Besides, intermittent fasting is a good way to control muscle mass, where they rise in the stomach. All this said the main reason people try to fast is fasting. We will discuss how intermittent fasting happens to get fat in a minute.

You need to understand that intermitted fasting is a strategy that you can use with ease and succeed in your endeavors. You do not have to opt to lift bad weights while maintaining good weight because it requires very little behavioral change. This is a good thing because it means that the fasting sequence falls into the category "simple and easy that you will do, but well enough that it can make a great difference. Have you tried various ways to get yourself in good shape only to end up disappointed? This book is critical to you because it contains all the information that you need to achieve your health goals. If you want to reduce weight, then you can be sure to get such benefits if you read and comprehend the information contained in this book. Let's get started!

Chapter 1: The Problem with Modern Diet

What Are Issues with Modern Diet?

We all know we need to eat healthily. We also know that we need to limit how much soda, drinks, processed foods, sugar we eat. But even though we know these things, it doesn't mean they are easy to follow.

According to a recent Food and Health Survey conducted by Psychology Today, 52 percent of Americans believe it is easier to calculate their taxes than know how to eat healthily. Too many people are having problems with this modern tax code, which means that many people have trouble figuring out how to eat the right foods for them.

We live in a country that is battling obesity. More than one-third of people in the United States are considered obese, and many are also considered to be overweight. However, these statistics do not show the full picture. Three out of three adults are considered overweight or obese, meaning that most people will fall into this category.

Why are these statistics so bad? Many factors contribute to obesity. One major culprit is classic American food. There has been a significant decline in the quality of our food as we have gone from a nation dependent on food from local farms to a nation that produces most of the food. This transition has increased our appetite for food because it is available now.

Also, many readily available and easily consumed foods are high in fat, sugar, and calories. All of these things help increase weight. From the sugary snacks, we get from the restroom to all the food chains around us, the quality of the food, and the amount we eat have dramatically changed. We can eat healthy foods without stopping if we want to, which is why obesity is so prevalent in our culture.

The first thing to look at is the amount of food we eat. The number of calories everyone needs may vary from person to person. Ingredients include your genes, your level of activity, your overall health, height, age, and gender. However, the target number used in food labels is about 2000 calories per day. This number is already fairly high for those living a stable life. It is also possible to eat 2000 calories or more in one sitting if you go out to eat.

Although the food out quickly us pushing the number of calories, it is also possible to eat too much when I eat at home. It is important to learn how to start eating what we need to work on, rather than eating because something tastes good, or we get bored, or tired.

To calculate the average daily calories consumed by Americans, organizations are examining the amount of food available per capita that shows the amount of food consumed. In the United States, this ends up around 3800 calories per day. Even when you take into account the fact that some of these foods are lost or discarded daily rather than eaten, the average American consumes 2700 calories per day. This is the approach that everyone will need, even if they lead an active lifestyle and not many Americans.

Now, we need to also discuss the quality of food most Americans eat. Growing up, most of us learn from our parents and teachers about what is good and what is not. Fruits and vegetables are seen as such well, and sugar and sweets are bad. The rest of the diet may not be as good as before, but they were good in moderation. Although we have been taught about healthy eating at an early age, it is still culturally difficult to follow these tips.

According to the Agricultural Department in the U.S., the top six sources of calories for most Americans are fruit-based sweets, yeast, poultry, sports/energy drinks, and alcoholic beverages. Remember that healthy fruits and vegetables are not listed. In the top five lists, the most common foods Americans eat are refined fruits and sugar. It is estimated that only 8% of the average American diet consists of fruits and vegetables.

According to a study by the US Department of Agriculture (USDA) in 2010, nuts, meat, and eggs make up 21% of these foods; oils and fats make up 23%, and calorie sweeteners make up 15%. Food that is not good for us constitutes 61 percent of our diet.

The time of day we eat is also important. Most Americans live a busy lifestyle and do not have time to sit and eat a balanced diet. In effect, they eat walking, usually in some areas unhealthy, or eat at night when their metabolism is slow. Besides, many Americans are sitting in bed and eating unhealthy snacks while watching television. Sometimes the diet is high, so we eat non-stop food.

It is important to learn the steps necessary to limit the amount of food we take each day. It is tempting to eat readily available foods. But, if you want to get back to your health and get better in a good way, it is important to stay away from classic American food and choose something good for you.

When you hear fasting, you can think of people who go for weeks without eating for religious reasons. You may think it is unhealthy or incapable of doing it because you love food. But intermittent fasting is different from religious fasting, although they share common ideas.

Indirect fasting is limiting your calorie intake in parts of the day or not eating too much on certain days. Your body still gets the nutrients it needs, but you eat fewer calories, so keeping it simple gravity. Some of the various types of fast cot will have discussed later in this book.

The reason this diet is successful is that it is effective in reducing the amount of fat in your body, as well as the number of calories you eat. Since you are reducing the time allowed to eat or reduce your calorie intake during certain days of the week, it is easy to lower your total calorie count. You can also choose how much time you would like to do quickly. Some people choose to do it for a month or more while others may fit their lifestyle, so they stick to it in the long run.

Avoid Unhealthy Eating Habits

After dinner, you are overweight, but you can't resist ordering desserts. If your stomach is hungry all day, then sweeten yourself until you fall asleep. Or maybe you can always eat something, such as walking, parking, or driving.

If any of these situations seem common, you can use your eating habits in preparation. They can all show unhealthy habits and can lose weight successfully for a long time.

Listen to Your Body

Anyone struggling with food allergies will develop a disruptive behavior that nutritionists can call. Poor eating habits can take many forms, from eating poorly to developing obesity and eating disorders, bulimia, or anorexia.

To allow yourself to want to lose weight and develop a healthy diet, your first step should be to accept your body and be proud that you are a member of a Weight Loss Program to keep your body healthy.

One of the best ways to regulate your eating habits is to stay active - learn how to eat when you are hungry and stop smoking after eating. It is easy to say, but with a little education, you will learn how to control your calories but not feel lost.

No One Is Perfect

Your goal should be to remain neutral, not perfect. Do not have physical cravings for food that can lead to physical inactivity, which can lead to many stomach ailments and eating disorders.

This book will help you improve your diet and create a diet plan that includes your favorite foods, including low-fat or healthy foods, to keep you healthy and satisfied. You need to slowly change your diet and improve your lifestyle to get the best results.

One powerful example to avoid eating is to put away a lot of calories from your face. Resistance is impossible when the food is under your nose!

But don't give up. You do not have to resist the urge to enter. What to do is to prevent parties and places with lots of junk food. Before you begin your first meal, please do a "stomach test": are you hungry, or do you just crave for something to eat?

If the food is like putting some oil in a container, our lives will be easier, but eating is more than an empty container.

Many cultural, behavioral, emotional, social, and environmental factors can help us determine how much time we spend in the stress of the job, and such hard experiences can make us start eating.
Consider whether you decide to eat or not, rather than decide without being conscious or unconscious. Can you choose what to eat? It will be easier if you start choosing a healthy diet - you will

have to regain the spirit as you experience the benefits of your tradition.

How to Change Bad Habits

Change is not always easy, especially for long-term behavior. So here are some tips to help you put away these bad habits into practice:

- Develop a plan to manage your daily contact with them. Decide how to address your weaknesses to be aware of the situation.
- Replace unhealthy foods with good food. If eating at night is your weakness, please give yourself a small snack in the evening.
- Too much sleep - it can slow down your eating time!
- Reduce TV viewing. You don't have time to try meals, and you have time to exercise.
- Set goals that are realistic for you. Not sure what will happen to you. Slowly change your habit of taking drugs.
- Thinking positive, negative thoughts like "I can't" or "I'm tired and distracted" can enable you to succeed in your course. Write inspirational ideas and read them when you need help to focus on your goals.
- Find your friends or hire supportive friends to maximize your chances of success. Studies have shown that support

is essential to the success of behavioral changes and barriers.

Brush Your Teeth After Dinner to Reduce the Temptation to Eat.

Foods buy organic foods (or personalized foods) that you can combine with fruit. The package that makes up the economy supports investing.

Wait at least ten minutes before seeking a second help to give your stomach time to express your thoughts. Eat your day with breakfast. According to one study, when most people eat calories in the morning, their total daily intake is less than calories in the evening.

Chapter 2: Intermitted Fasting, What Is It?

What does the actual meaning of fasting mean? Almost all of us know the word fast. The reasons people quickly differ are from one group to another. For some people, it is a religious tradition; they sacrifice to pray. Others have no reason to; they just eat food. In early societies, people used to go to the woods to work and to eat while they rest.

Temporary fasting is not part of the fasting practices described above. It is not a religious tradition, nor does it drive without time and no food - it is an option. It is best described as a diet pattern that changes during meal times and fasting periods, with each season running at a fixed time. For example, in the 16:8 type, you fast 16 hours and 8 hours when you can eat.

Note that it is not food but a form of eating. Less is said about the foods you should eat, but more emphasis is placed on eating. Does this mean you can eat anything you want? The truth is you mat eat what you want. Like everything else in life, you will need to get out of what you are into. Eating clean is one of the three factors in the success of a successful diet. Does this mean you live with chicken and broccoli? We are human beings and believe in enjoying life, but as you already know, moderation is the key here.

It is important to note that IF is not a program that is out of place, will change over time, and disappear like most weight loss programs. It has been around for a long time and has been popular for many years (even now you are learning it). It is one of the first health and fitness changes in the world today, and it is recommended by a variety of health and fitness experts.

Intermittent Fasting History

When you compare the traditional "diet," fasting is easier and less stressful. It is always done. You know that you will be conscious every time you don't eat breakfast or dinner. Historically, our ancestors were fasting during the hunting season.

Once the field is established, civilization will follow. If there is not enough food or season, people will fast without problems. Cities and fortresses process cereals and meat in the winter. Before watering, no rain means famine. People should store food for as long as possible before fasting until the rain returns, and the crop can be revived.

Religion develops in this way of living together, sharing, and spreading beliefs and customs. Religion also records fasting.

Hindus call it "Vaasa" and designate special days or holidays, using personal pens or commemorating their gods. Islam and Judaism have Ramadan and Yom Kippur, which is a place where work, food, clothes, and love are forbidden. In the Catholic Church, fast six weeks before Easter or Holy Week.

Fasting Science

Modern agriculture and the "food" industry (or food-like things) have completely changed the way people view or eat food every day, leading to the laundry list that today's society faces. IF is an ancient tradition, and the science behind its health benefits will soon be available to the public. When fasting, you can basically make your body clean, repair, and restore its best function.

The three main health promotion methods associated with fasting include biological metabolic control, glandular dysfunction, and various lifestyles.

Circadian Rhythm Biology

Humans (and other organisms) have evolved into biological clocks that produce circadian rhythms to ensure that your body functions work in a negative time throughout the day.

They occur in a 24-hour light-dark cycle and are affected by biological and behavioral changes.

Body fluid consumption can negatively affect metabolism, which may lead to being overweight and diseases like cancer, heart disease, and type 2 diabetes.

This Is a Place for Temporary Fasting.

Eating symptoms seems to be the main time for how your body works and regulates metabolism, physiology, and behavioral ways that contribute to your overall health and well-being.

Certain behavioral interventions, such as (you guessed it!) indirect fasting, can promote the synthesis of circadian rhythms, leading to gene expression, metabolism, and changes in hormones and weight control, all of which play an important role in your health result.

Microbiome of the Gut Microbiome

The gastrointestinal tract (GI), also known as the intestine, plays a very important role in regulating multiple processes in the body.

Many bowel movements (and almost all physical and biological activities in the body) are affected by the above-mentioned circadian rhythm.

For example, gastric emptying during the day, blood flow and glucose metabolism are more frequent than at night.

Therefore, chronic obstructive pulmonary edema may affect bowel function, leading to an increased risk of poor metabolism and chronic disease.

The gut microbiome, also known as our "second brain," has become a broad target for health and disease research because of its wide participation in the body's metabolism, physiology, nutrition, and prevention.

Direct fasting has a direct and positive impact on the disease microbiome:

Slow down

- Insufficient system structure
- Promote energy balance by strengthening self-esteem
- With a great understanding of the potential for disease prevention and treatment, research on bowel and fasting is still emerging.

Life Behavior

Intermittent fasting has been shown to alter various health behaviors such as calorie intake (e.g., how much you eat), energy expenditure (when you are exercising), and sleep.

No wonder these three factors are one of the biggest factors in fasting today: losing weight.

A recent study showed that increasing the fasting time at night to more than 14 hours resulted in a significant reduction in calorie intake and weight gain due to:

- Energy level
- Sleep satisfaction
- Sleep restrictions

Intermittent fasting also reduces nighttime eating, which leads to poor sleep quality and reduced sleep time, leading to increased insulin resistance and obesity, diabetes, heart disease, and cancer.

The next question you might encounter is why you should consider fasting first. Humans have experienced fasting for many years. Sometimes they do this because it is necessary because they can't afford anything. Then there is time to fast for religious reasons. Religions such as Buddhism, Christianity, and

Islam advocate some form of fasting. Fasting is also normal when you are sick.

Although fasting sometimes has a negative meaning, fasting does not have any natural meaning. Our bodies are better able to cope with the time we should not eat. Many things in the body change when we are fasting. This will help our body stay active during the drought.

When we fast, we find a significant decrease in insulin and blood sugar levels, and also an improved increase in Human Growth Hormone. Although it was done in the early stages of food shortages, it was used to help people lose weight. Burning fat becomes lighter, easier, and more effective.
Some people decide to go faster because it helps their metabolism. This fasting is good for correcting various health problems. There is also evidence that regular fasting can help you live longer. Studies have shown that these mice live longer in the fasting zone.

Other studies have shown that fasting can prevent various diseases such as Alzheimer's disease, cancer, type 2 diabetes, and heart disease. Then some people choose to go faster because it suits their lifestyle. Fasting is helpful for life. For example, the less food you have to do, the easier it will be to live.

Why Do You Want to Fast?

Intermittent fasting is a practice of diet planning so that your body can get the most out of it. Fasting is a simple, sensible, and healthy way to promote weight loss, rather than reducing calorie intake by eliminating all your favorite foods or maintaining a normal diet. There are many ways to fast, but it is defined as a specific diet. This model focuses on the transformations you make while eating, not what you eat.

When you start with an intermittent fast, you are likely to keep your calories the same, but instead of spreading your food throughout the day, you will eat larger meals over a shorter period. For example, instead of eating 3 to 4 meals a day, you can eat one large meal at 11 am, and then another large meal at 6 pm, with no food between 11 am and 6 pm, and 6 -After the evening, eat until 11 am. This is one way of fasting, and others will be discussed in this book in later chapters. However, you must first understand why this method works.

Intermittent fasting is a method used by many bodybuilders, athletes, and members of the body to gain muscle mass and percentage of body fat low. It's a simple strategy that allows you to eat your favorite foods while still promoting fat loss and muscle gain or maintenance. Endless fasting can be applied in a short or long time, but the best results come from adopting this lifestyle in your daily life.

While the word "fasting" can intimidate the average person, indirect fasting does not mean that your soul is hungry. To understand the managers behind the successful transition zone, we first go through the two digestive regions of the region: the feeding region and the fasting region. Three to five hours after eating, your body is in what is called the "fed state." During the feeding phase, your insulin levels increase to absorb and balance your diet. With increased insulin levels, it is not easy for the body to burn fast. Insulin is a hormone produced by the pancreas to regulate the levels of glucose in the blood. Despite its purpose for regulating, insulin is technically a storage hormone. When your insulin levels are high, your body burns your food for energy rather than your stored fat, which is why increased levels prevent weight loss.

After three to five hours are full, your body has completed the meal preparation, and you enter the recovery state. The condition behind absorption lasts from 8 to 12 hours. This time the difference is when your body enters the fasting state. Since your body has completely processed your diet at this time, your insulin levels are low, making the stored fat more likely to burn. Fasting state, your body does not have the energy left to eat, so reserves are burned. Regular fasting allows your body to achieve the fat-burning rate that you would normally achieve on an average, 'three meals a day' mode of eating. This alone is why many people experience immediate results without intermittent fasting without even altering their physical activity while eating, or eating. They simply change the timing and the way they eat.

When you start the program for fast and relentless, it may take some time to leave things out. Don't be discouraged! If you change, get back to the fast mode when you can. Avoid hitting yourself or feeling guilty. Negative self-esteem goes a long way in getting back into your shape. Making a lifestyle change takes a conscious effort, and no one expects to do it right away. Unless it is known that you are going for a long time. Since when you eat, fast and relentless you will take some time to learn. As soon as you choose the right course for you, focus and be positive, you will find your place in no time.

Unlike some of the other meal plans, you may have to continue; fasting will work. It uses your body and how it works to its advantage to help you lose weight. It's easy to hear some fear when fasting. You can assume that you need to live for days and weeks without eating (and being able to put off their diet for a long time even when they want to lose weight), and it will be difficult for you.

Fasting endless slightly different from the one you think you can. Not only is it really difficult to fast for weeks at a time, but it is also not good for the body. Your body will often go into a state of hunger if you eventually fast. It will take you to spend a lot of time without eating so the body will work to save calories and help you keep up with fat and calories as long as possible. This means you will not only be hungry but also lose weight.

You do not have to worry about how fast fasting will work in the process of starvation. Fasting is effective because you will not be fasting until the body gets into this state of hunger and stops losing weight. In hindsight, it makes fasting long enough for you to be able to speed up your metabolism.

With a temporary fast, you will find that when you go for a few hours without eating (usually no more than 24 hours), the body will not go straight into the hunger process. Instead, it wants to eliminate available calories. If you ate the right amount of calories during the day, the body will return to eating until it consumes the stored fat deposits and uses it as fuel. Likewise, when you follow a series of fasting plans, you force your body to burn more fat without putting in any extra work.

Here are some quick tips for success:

First and foremost, you mustn't expect to see results from your new lifestyle immediately. In effect, you need to plan on doing the task at least 30 days before you start judging the results correctly. Second, it is important to keep in mind that the quality of the food you put into your body is still important as it only takes a few quick meals to finish all your hard work. Finally, for the best results, you will need to incorporate a simple exercise routine during the fasting days and a more gentle exercise on full-calorie days.

Intermittent Fasting Types

Several major types of intermittent fasting are there that you can choose to follow. These Somalis can all be effective, and the one that suits you will depend on your preferences, your schedule, and your lifestyle. Some of the fasting options you can go with include:

- Method 16/8: This will ask you to fast 16 hours daily and eat for the other 8 hours. So, you can choose to eat only from noon until 8 pm or after 10 pm. You can choose one of your favorite eight-hour windows.

- Eat-Eat: In a week, it could be twice or once when you will not consume anything from the first day to the next. This gives you a 24-hour fast but still allows you to eat every day of your fast.

- 5: 2: You will choose two days of the week to fast. During those two days, you are only allowed to have up to 500-600 calories per day.

Of course, there are differences between the three above. For example, some people decide to limit their even bigger windows by eating only four hours and fasting for this fast. Most people who fast this fast choose to follow the 16/8 method because it is the easiest to adapt and will give you great results along the way. The fasting is simple and effective. It helps you to limit the calories you eat and burn more fats and calories than you normally feed.

Chapter 3: How Do You Fast?

One thing that many people like about interactive fasting is that it can offer you many options. As I mentioned, there are several different ways you can do a quick fix based on your schedule and lifestyle. Some people find that they have a few busy days during the week and so those days will fast. Others like the idea of reducing their eating window and doing fasting every day.

The fasting method you choose is yours. They can all be very effective and will give you some of the benefits you are looking for. Let's look at some of the fasting options you can go with, so you can choose the one that is right for you.

The 16:8 Method

There are different ways to learn IF. However, they all have the same meaning; all are in seasonal feeding and fasting.

- The time to fast – it depends on the time length in different methods. During this time, you have not eaten at all or zero-calorie drinks.

- Feeding time – also varies with the length of time in each method. During this time, you can eat whatever you want moderately to avoid too many drinks. It is advisable to eat normally and do not look like compensation during your lack of food. Some features like Warrior Diet may require you to eat foods in a particular way.

Before we look at the 16: 8 method, it is important to point out that temporary fasting is not for everyone. Below are some of the people who can't try the temporary fast:

- Under People under 18 years
- People with diabetes (both type 1 and 2) without seeing a doctor first
- Mothers Pregnant and lactating mothers
- People with Eating Disorders
- People with low body fat
- People with high cortisol levels

WARNING: Before you do any diet, exercise program or your usual changes should go to a doctor or other relevant professional.

Now let's look at the 16: 8 method in particular.

16:8 Schedule

As the name implies, this method is divided into two periods; for 16 hours of fasting and 8 hours of feeding time. It is important to monitor your feeding time regularly. This means that you cannot decide to eat from 8 am to 4 pm today and change from 8 pm to 4 am the next day. This is designed to create a schedule that is easy for your body to adapt to and easy to follow. Remember, the hungry hormones are released concerning eating habits? Changing your routine regularly will make you hungry all the time and experience a problem with these hormones.

This method is said to be durable and easy to stick to as you are not required to live without food for a long time, and can easily adapt to the lives of most people in everyday life. For example, the average person sleeps for eight hours. You only need to fast for an additional 8 hours while you are awake, making the fasting period shorter.

For example, if your last meal was at 10 pm, you would fast until 2 pm the next day, and some would sleep, while others would be busy - you won't know exactly when. This method is popular as you can still have dinner with your family or friends before your feeding window closes. Important note: Some research suggests eating late at night produces higher insulin than daytime affects sleep quality and enhances nighttime storage.

Factors to Consider for Achieving Success

Goal Setting

I recommend that you have a clear view of what you want to achieve. Not as many goals as I want to get - "fit," "healthy," or "lose two pounds" just won't cut it when it's hard. You need a clear reason to do this, or you are likely to quit. When I train a client, I tell them to consider 3 things.

What do you want to do that you cannot currently attend?
- 30 days
- 90 days
- 12 Months

What do you want to look like?
- 30 days
- 90 days
- 12 Months

How do you want to feel?
- 30 days
- 90 days
- 12 Months

When they complete this, I also tell them to ask themselves why they want these things and what they think will be different from these goals. This will help you identify what matters to you. Many times our goals originate from external influences, but at the end of the day, they should be right for you. Analyze your data and set:

- Day Goal
- Day Goal
- Month Goal

Collection

Evaluate your schedule! I always see people who choose only the dining window, so I have time to eat during this time. Not a good start! Also, assess where you might struggle to go without food. For example, if you are a lazy mocker it is not wise to set your fasting window during the slowest part of your day. If eating dinner with your family is a tradition, then allow your dining window. Be smart when choosing a feeder window. Make this task as easy as possible for yourself.

Support

It is important to surround yourself with good people on the same journey. It will be difficult, and in some cases, you will need to stop. Finding other people to support you is the key to success and can be the difference between quitting and continuing!

Maintain Discipline

Of all the things you can find in the world, discipline is one of the most valuable. Discipline is the most important factor you need to have long-term success. Even though you may be fasting and losing weight, there is a huge burden on discipline because you have to actively train your mind and not want the body's diet. In most cases, people allow their physical desires to take over and make their own decisions.

When you fast, you actively seek discipline to make sure you do not let your body make the decisions for you.

When you can continue discipline, this has an impact on your entire life. When you choose to urinate on what you love, this will eventually lead to your demise.

Patience Pays

It is often proved that patience is good. When you can be patient, you can endure and weather any difficult situation with the knowledge that you will overcome the other.

The opposite of a sick person is that of angry anger. Anger is usually associated with children. Importantly, an adult can be easily seen as an adult because when they do not find their way quickly, they throw a fit.

When you are working toward a goal like stress, there will be some negatives involved. This does not mean that you will never be able to be satisfied. It means you can't have an item right away.

When you can actively participate in the rejection of yourself temporarily because of a specific goal, you will be able to apply that virtue to other aspects of your life.

Have a Clear Mind

In many cases, people share the power of fasting with the evidence of their minds. Many people go through stress and anxiety. When you can get rid of these points, this will help you to focus specifically. This is because you have no fog associated with the brain.

When your mind is clear, you will be able to think in a way that is physically perfect for what you want.

When your mind is stressed with anxiety, you will make decisions that are not always the best. Those decisions do not reflect what you want deeply because fear affects you.

When your mind is clear, you eliminate issues like fear, anxiety, and depression.
Understand the power of the mind. Wherever your mind goes, your life will follow. When you can prove something, you will be able to have a completely different experience but with more power.

Effective Reliability

For centuries, fasting has been recognized as a major component of certain religious groups. It is famous for Islam, Judaism, and Christianity. Most people who practice fasting practice at certain times of the year (Ramadan, Rent, etc.). At these times, they eliminate something they especially want (food, TV, social media) to focus their attention on God.

When deciding to fast weight loss purposes, you may feel a little bit different. However, if you maintain a spiritual belief in a higher power, this will affect that relationship. This is because you may be able to rely on something superior to help you withstand your body tests.

This culture is especially good for people who are emotionally eating to cope with their emotions. When you do not have the food you have in your hands, this forces you to rely on the higher power (religious or not) to get the strength you need to overcome difficult times.

Confidence

In most cases, people do not allow themselves to develop the strength that is really within them.

- When you can work out your self-denial fasting, this is a confidence boost.
- When you can check out something on your list of activities that is difficult, this will make you feel good about yourself and your abilities.
- When you know you can overcome something difficult, this changes the way you view yourself.

It also affects how you view future challenges. When you can overcome a challenge, it gives you the confidence to continue. When you feel mentally strong, this will affect your ability to look at the situation rather than the situation, and you will come out with the challenge.

Resetting

There are times when people are constantly eating and not having time to give up. When you fast for weight loss, this is a good opportunity to get rehab.

You are allowed to clean your system and get rid of any problems. This is not just physical. This is from a psychological and spiritual perspective, as well.

If you like proverbial resettlement, many people do the same when the holidays are over. During the holidays, people eat and drink because it is a popular season. However, it may not common for individuals to have an overwhelming feeling after it is over.

This is one of the main reasons people start weight loss trips as a New Year's resolution. For many, it is an attempt to repair or delay the process.

Productivity

There are many different types of articles, videos, and all where people like to discuss life create more productive. Maintaining high levels of productivity is to achieve great success in the eyes of many. While this may not be important to everyone, many people believe this.

As a result, many people are looking for ways to increase their productivity to make them feel successful. If you would like to enjoy the added benefit of fasting, understand that productivity can fall under this umbrella. This is mainly because production can be a clear product.

When you are focused and do not have the burden of stress on your brain, this naturally increases your ability to produce more. Consider how you feel after eating Thanksgiving. In most cases, people return to tiredness and the length of the bed near you. While the body takes time to digest all these foods, it will spend more energy on your efforts to complete other tasks. As a result, people are slow and want to sleep.

If you fast, your body does not spend as much energy to digest it except water. As a result, you have more energy to engage in other activities.

Rest

One of the benefits of fasting for weight loss is the ability to relax and relax. When your mind is clear, and you will not be dealing with too much stress, this will help you remain in a state of mind for a long time. So, when you sleep, it will be easier for you to avoid falling asleep.

This is great news for people struggling with insomnia or sleep issues. As you develop a nighttime routine and are in the middle of fasting, your body will be able to turn around and have an easy time getting quality rest.

Tips to Help You Sleep Well

Get Enough Sunlight

Our body system or "body clock" plays an important role in producing hormones. This is strongly influenced by sunlight. Stevenson explained that Light, especially sunlight, signals your glands and organs to be the time to wake up, waiting in line to produce the hormones of the day (often helping you stay alert and awake). If our body receives less sunlight and more light in the morning (such as televisions, laptops, and smartphones), our circadian clock will rise. This can cause our glands to produce hormones that prevent them from falling asleep. Poor quality of sleep hinders the production of hormones such as HGH and can even stimulate the production of hormones such as insulin. If that happens, we will not burn fat at night!

Avoid Watching Before You Go to Bed

If you are watching TV until 11 pm or sleeping on your phone, the quickest way to improve sleep is to stop using your device at least an hour before bedtime. Remember how our body clock affects sunlight? It is also influenced by artificial light. Our eyes are great light sensors, and the blue light emitted by our favorite screen stimulates our body to produce day-to-day hormones and primarily makes us awake and active. For these bad boys in our body, insomnia will be difficult, and our bodies will not produce the anabolic hormones we need to repair and lose weight. Some of Stevenson's evidence only came out in the dark. Have fun!

Some people often argue that watching television or other device helps them sleep without being distracted. The above information is to achieve quality sleep, and although you may feel it, I find it in most cases, this is because the client has made it a habit. I encourage you to find other activities to change your equipment, rather than lying in the dark about worrying about not going to sleep.

Dark Sleep

While this may seem obvious after the first two tips, some people forget this guide when they were not told. We cannot control outdoor lights, such as traffic lights and disturbing safety lights, but these can still affect our sleep at the molecular level, interrupting maintenance, and making us tired the next day. Leave your windows with heavy curtains to stop the fog outside of the lights that are damaging your healing process!

Quality Is Not Quantity

One of the most useful points I have come across in Stevenson's book is that there is a window of sweet time during the night where sleep is the most effective. During this window, our body produces the highest number of hormones needed for repair and fat loss. He explained that this was about 10 pm to 2 am and clock out the window. He also noted that this can vary depending on the time of year and the time you are in, but he advised that you get to bed as soon as possible after dark.

Improving your sleep habits is the key to weight loss, muscle building, and living a healthier life in general. This important ingredient is often overlooked in weight loss programs and maybe the remaining part you need! Proper sleep will ensure the adaptation of the essential hormone to fat-burning maybe even more important than increasing your exercise habits. Set a regular bedtime and make sure you lie in bed about 30 to 60 minutes ahead.

Power

When you have power, you have resilience. When you endure, nothing can stop your path. The advantages of fasting to lose weight include your ability to improve. When you are working on developing talent, it is a good idea to start small.

Think about fasting for specific hours a day. So, as you manage those goals, build on that for many hours. A long time ago, you will be able to do three days of fasting without much difficulty. When you can fast for a long time, this will increase endurance and ability.

Stay Strong

One of the reasons people love superheroes is because of their strength. They can force them when they need to achieve a goal.

Although the superheroes of their weakness, they can find ways of overcoming. When you can fast for weight loss and lose weight, this will allow you to develop an inner strength that you can apply to your spiritual, personal, and professional life.

No matter, know that it has many benefits for fasting. Don't trust the hype when people say that fasting is dangerous.

When you do it right, it can directly impact your entire life and make you a better person. Even though you are fasting for weight loss, your mind and body will improve your life significantly.

Try to Avoid Your Temptation.

One thing that may hinder your efforts on fasting days is the temptation of other foods in your cupboard. If you are fairly sensitive to visual experimenting with food, you may need to shop every few days instead of shopping every week or two. It can also help if you have family members or someone who lives with you and will not follow Fasting.

Prepare Your Refrigerator to Make Fasting Days Easier.

Try to place your food on the fasting day on the refrigerator shelf. This can help train your eyes (and your mind) that only those foods are available on fasting days. Eventually, you may find that your eyes are not wandering around in the fridge, looking at foods you can't eat.

Remember That Social Meeting Does Not Have to Be Included in Food.

Eating out can be a big part of your social life. Sharing a good meal or several drinks with friends and family is part of our culture. However, there are many other things you can do to enjoy the fasting days that do not involve eating. Focusing on these activities will help keep your mind away from food but will ensure that you do not become a vet when fasting. Invite some friends to go to a tennis game, take an art show, spend a day at the beach, or sign up for a dance class with a bill.

If You Are a Sanitizer, Stay Away from the Triggers.

Many of us have stimulants, except at mealtimes or hunger, which shows us to eat. Time off work can be automatically sent to us by a vending machine. Watching TV can be adapted to mealtimes. You may want to bring the leftovers to your children when you clean the dishes. Spend some time before your meal is listed at mealtimes, and then make a plan to deal with these triggers while eating. Take time off from work and have the opportunity to take a ten-minute walk. Allow other family members to clean the plates after dinner. Make work needles, cut cards or cabbage, do some extension, or chew gum when you are watching television.

Reward Yourself

The best way to achieve a great goal is to set a few small ones and celebrate them as they have achieved them. For any of the days of fasting completed or any lost pounds, treat yourself a little. It can be weights, a new book, an evening out with you and your husband, or just an hour to yourself.

Learn to Tell the Difference Between Hunger and Other Emotions.

Most of us eat junk food. We eat because we are angry, we eat because we are not lazy, or we eat because we are tired. Begin writing down your feelings when you are thinking about taking a snack. You may find that most of the time, you just need to move, talk on the phone with a friend, or go to sleep.

If you feel hungry, drink water.

It is often difficult to tell the difference between thirst and hunger. Each time you feel a craving for a snack, drink a glass of water. You may find that hunger pangs often disappear.

Other Ways of Intermittent Fasting

Diet 5:2

Another option you can go with is the 5:2 diet. This one asks you to eat in a normal manner for five days of the week with the discipline to limit yourself to no more than 600 calories the other two days. This is sometimes called the "fasting" as well.

Nowadays fast, it is recommended that women should stay at 500 calories and 600 calories for men. For example, you will eat normally every day of the week, and on Monday and Thursday, you will only eat two small meals for a total of 500-600 calories. You can choose any day of the week like the days of fasting until you do not put them back. Choose the two busiest days of the week and do your fasting.

There aren't many studies out there about the 5:2 diet, but since it's fast, it will give you the many benefits you are looking for. You will be able to do it without having to worry about making food all day.

Eat a Regular Diet

Diet-Eating requires you to avoid eating 24 hours once or twice a week. This model was first published by Brad Pilon and was a popular way to do it consistently over a while. It is possible to fast in the fast while still eating one meal a day. Most people eat dinner after day and do not eat until after dinner the next day. This will allow you to never go for a whole day without eating but fail during the 24-hour drinking period.

You can change this however you like. If you find it easier to skip breakfast or lunch or lunch to lunch, then you can choose one of these options. During your fasting, you are allowed to have coffee, water, and other calorie-free beverages to satisfy yourself, but you are not allowed to have any food at all.

Remember that you only fast for one or two days a week. When it is time to eat normally, you need to eat the same food that you would have if you were not fasting. This will help you lose weight without damaging your body.

The main issue of continuing such a fast is the 24-hour fast is difficult for most people. However, you can easily. You may find that starting with a fast, such as a 16-hour fast, can give you better results, and then you can start fasting longer. Going all day without eating can be difficult, and most people choose to follow one of the other fasting options to see the same results.

Another Fasting Day

With this option, you will be fasting every other day. There are several options you can go with, and it will depend on what works for your needs. Some fasting allows you to have around

500 calories in your fasting days. You will find that most laboratory studies about the transition zone used some form of fasting day to assist in determining all the health benefits.

Fasting every other day can be difficult for most people. Forcing you to fast every other day can be a challenge. Fasting every other day is something you will need to build on. You are likely to feel hungry several times a week for fasting, and it is difficult to cope in the long run.

Worrier Food

This is another popular option that you can choose from during non-stop fasting. It involves eating small quantities of raw fruits and vegetables during the day, followed by plenty of evening meals. This requires you to fast throughout the day, to eat enough to satisfy, and to eat in the four-hour window at night.

This food is one of the first foods to incorporate some kind of indirect fasting. Such diets also include food choices similar to Paleo food. You will not fast most of the day and night celebrations, but you will be eating a diet full of foods that look like what you can discover in nature.

Skipping Meals Spontaneously

You can try this if you want to prepare your body for a temporary fast or if you don't want to worry too much when eating. In this zone, you do not need to worry about following one of the more structured fasting plans. From time to time, you will skip meals. You can do this when you are hungry or when you are busy and not eating. It is a great myth that you have to eat every hour to avoid starvation.

The body adapts well to dealing with a long time without eating. It lacks a number of foods, especially if you are not hungry or busy; it does not harm your body. Every time you skip a meal or two, you do it technically. If you are too busy to have breakfast at the door, make sure you eat a healthy lunch and dinner. If you miss work assignments and are unable to find a place to eat, then it is okay to miss out on food. This is not harmful, and it really helps to save time.

You may not see good results compared to some of the other options, but it is better than nothing and easy to work with. You may try to skip a meal or two during the week and lose some weight when it works. As you can see, there are many different options that you can work with when you are ready to go fasting. Some of these will be easier than others, and some may fit your schedule better. You will need to choose the fastest way to work in your daily life.

Chapter 4: Why Should You Do Intermittent Fasting?

There are various plans for meals that you can choose. Some will help you limit your carbon intake and focus on good fats and protein. Some will limit your fat intake and focus on a healthy, healthy scourge.

With all the options on the market and a few of them being legitimate weight loss options, you need to know why you need to be fast and uninterrupted. This unit will look at the various benefits of direct fasting and how it will change your health.

It Modulates the Cells, Hormones and Genes Function

The failure to eat for a while leads to certain things happening to the body. For instance, it will start to regulate cell function and change some of your hormone levels, making it easier for body fat to enter. Other changes that may occur in the body include:

- Levels of insulin: insulin levels will decline slightly, which makes it easier for the body to burn fat.

- Human Growth Hormone: Growth hormone blood level can significantly increase. High levels of this hormone can help build muscle and burn fat.
- Cell Repair: The body will begin the process of repairing the cells, such as removing the waste from all the cells
- Genetic profiling: Some beneficial mutations occur in several genes that will help you live longer and protect against disease.

Weight Loss and Body Fat

Many people go fast in succession to lose weight. In most cases, indirect fasting will naturally help you eat less. You will end up consuming fewer calories, which will lead to weight loss. Besides, fasting strengthens the hormone to facilitate weight loss. Low growth hormone and insulin levels help your body break down fat and use energy. This is why short-term fasting can increase your metabolism by at least three percent.

On the one hand, it boosts your metabolism to burn more calories while also reducing the amount you eat. According to a review that was released in 2014concerning the scientific studies of intermittent fasting, people were able to lose up to 8 percent of their body weight in less than 24 weeks.

It Helps with Diabetes

Type 2 diabetes is a disease that has become popular in recent years. Anything that could lower the resistance of insulin could also be useful in lowering the blood sugar levels hence protecting you from type 2 diabetes.

According to some researches on Intermittent Fasting, there was a reduction of blood sugar from three to six percent, while insulin was reduced by 21 percent and 31 percent. A study carried on rats that were diabetic also proved that Intermittent Fasting could be crucial in the protection of rats from kidney damage; a common challenge for diabetics. This suggests that indirect fasting may be a good option for people at high risk for type 2 diabetes.

Simplifying Life

While this may not be considered a health benefit like any other, it is still important to note. Many people find that temporary fasting can make life easier. They know that they need to have a focus on to eat, as long as they are allowed to eat for hours. They can go a few days a week without having to worry about eating. Overall, this meal plan can make your life easier.

When you can cut down on some of the work you need to do during the day and focus on something else, you may end up worrying about your life. We all know that stress can hurt our health and our lives. When you can reduce stress, it is easy to be the healthiest version of yourself.

Good on the Heart

Heart disease is considered to be the world's largest killer. Intermittent fasting can help with some of these risk factors, such as low blood sugar levels, inflammatory markers, blood triglycerides, cholesterol, and high blood pressure. The main issue is that many studies on intermittent fasting have been conducted in animals. We need to do more studies that test fasting and human heart health.

Can Help with Cancer

Many people get cancer every year. This disease can lead to extreme conditions, and its characteristics include cells growing in an uncontrolled manner. Fasting is something that is said to be having great benefits in terms of your metabolism, which can lead to a reduction in cancer risk. Some human studies show that fasting cancer patients have been able to alleviate some of the chemical side effects.

Good on the Mind

Something considered to be working for the physical body could also work for the brain? Fasting can help improve the metabolic symptoms that are common in helping the brain stay healthy as well. This may include helping with insulin resistance, lowering blood sugar levels, reduced inflammation, and chemical stress.

There have been several studies conducted in rats showing how intermittent fasting can contribute to the growth of nerve cells, which improves brain function. Fasting can also help to increase the levels of brain activity that arise. When the brain is deficient in this, it can cause depression as well as other mental issues.

It Helps to Improve Cells

When we move fast, human cells can begin to be called the "resistance" of the digestive process. This involves breaking down the cells and metabolizing any proteins that are no longer used. As self-medication increases, it can help prevent human illnesses like cancer and Alzheimer's disease.

May Prevent Alzheimer's Disease

Alzheimer's is a neurological disease that has become common nowadays. The disease is not curable, and to ensure you are safe from it, prevention is better than cure. According to a particular study which was contacted on rats, one of the ways to prevent the disease is through intermittent fasting.

There are some cases whereby findings suggest that if you include fasting on a daily basis can have a positive impact when it comes to dealing with Alzheimer's disease. The studies have been done to both animals and human beings. Apart from this disease the studies also indicate that intermittent fasting can help in the prevention of other diseases like Parkinson's and Huntington diseases

Some case reports indicate that lifestyle changes (including daily or at least short-term fasting) help improve the symptoms of Alzheimer's disease in nine of the 10 patients. Animal studies have also shown that this fasting can help prevent other neurological diseases such as Huntington's disease and Parkinson's disease.

Although most of these studies were done on animals, the results seemed promising. Temporary fasting is a trend, and research on its mechanisms for good health is not new. It takes time to learn all the benefits of fasting.

Regular Fasting Can Help You Live Longer

One of the most interesting things about interactive fasting is that it can help you live longer. Several studies in rodents have shown how intermittent fasting can help extend their lifespan—similar to what happens when you gradually reach the regular calorie limit. In some studies, the effect was surprisingly low. One is that animals that fast every day live 83% more than those that do not.

While it is difficult to justify an increase in its lifespan due to the intermittent fasting still has not been conducted in research on long-term populations to determine this, it is still a popular idea for those trying to prevent aging. Given the known benefits of the metabolism of this diet, it is no wonder that people believe that regular fasting will help them stay alive and healthy.

As you can see, there are many benefits to following a fast-food diet. We have only touched on a few of them, but there have been many studies on the effects of this diet and why it may be useful for you. If you are trying to improve your mental health, live longer, lose weight, or gain more energy, indirect fasting can improve your life.

Issues Associated with Being Overweight

The kidneys work to clean the blood, removing impurities and water through the urine. It helps regulate blood pressure, which keeps the body healthy and active. When the kidneys are injured, and they cannot filter the blood as it is called kidney disease. When the filter is not right, the waste can build up in the body. Too much fat increases blood pressure and diabetes which is one of the major causes of kidney disease. According to recent studies, even when the condition is not present, obesity can directly cause kidney disease, especially if uncontrolled.

Diseases of Behavior

Steatohepatitis (non-alcoholic steatohepatitis (NASH)) also called fatty liver disease, occurs due to fat formation in the liver, which causes damage. This fatty liver can cause a number of injuries including liver failure, cirrhosis (tumor tissue), severe liver damage, etc. Occasionally, fatty liver disease may not permit the symptoms of an illness such as hepatitis B but not as a result of excessive drinking.

Osteoarthritis

Osteoarthritis is a health problem that causes pain and stiffness in the joints. This health issue is always related to age and injury. It usually affects the bones in the lower back, the waist, the knees, and the hands. Obesity is one of the common risk factors for developing osteoarthritis. Other factors include heredity, aging, and injury.

More pressure is put on the joints due to the extra weight. The bones and joints covered in fibrous tissue become tired due to the pressure of the fat and body weight. Also, high body fat can mean dangerous substances in the blood that may increase the risk of inflammation.

Sleep Apnea

One or more shortness of breath produces this problem when you are asleep. People with this condition can have heart failure, focusing on difficulty and daytime sleepiness. According to research, sleep deprivation can be caused by obesity. This is because a person with a lot of fat around their neck may have fewer airways. In fact, small airways can cause difficulty in breathing, or breathing can be very loud, often referred to as shortness of breath. In chronic cases, breathing can stop for a while before it can continue. Also, fat stored in the neck can increase the risk of inflammation caused by sleep apnea.

Stroke

When the flow of blood to the brain stops, there are high chances of experiencing a stroke. When this happens, it means that one may get ischemic stroke because of the blockage of the blood that flows to the brain. Sometimes one may experience another type of stroke called Hemorrhagic, which happens due to the rapturing of blood vessels. When blood pressure increases because of obesity or obesity, stabbing is more likely. Other problems commonly associated with strokes include heart disease, high blood sugar, and high cholesterol.

Understanding Your Body and Intermittent Fasting

Before you begin with any periodic fasting program, you need to fully understand your plan and know if it will go down well with your body type or not. Adjusting your portions or how often you eat may work better than occasional fasting. No two people will respond to a set of incentives in the same way. So you choose the one that works best for you.

Want to give it a shot? Then dip your toe in the water to feel it. Go all day fasting without eating a bite. There is no problem. You will feel very uncomfortable, and you will have a lot of empathy. At this point, you will want to throw in the towel and leave. Your productivity may decrease, headaches, and other symptoms may begin within a few hours after remembering to eat. If you are strong enough to handle this and decide to go ahead with the program, where do you set up your tent? Just go through the types of fasting listed and figure out which one works best for you. You should also know that fasting can be done permanently or stopped when the desired weight is obtained. To keep in touch with how much weight you have lost, keep track of your calorie intake, fasting times, and your weight for longer.

Cleaning System

You can always come up with your own fasting program with ay features included in other fasting programs. To do this, however, make sure you are not new to the whole process. To build your plan, here are a few tips to have in the back of your mind.

- All programs have features called mealtimes and fasting times.
- The time you eat is much shorter than the last time.
- Make sure you do not go into starvation mode, which starts about 38 hours of food insecurity. The maximum allowable fasting time is 24 hours. Anything after this contradicts itself.

The Journey to Having a Successful Fasting Program Can Be Very Difficult.

Here are some guidelines to help you get through the field.

- Take it one step at a time to understand what the program covers. Try a little fasting program. You don't want to jump first into something he or she may have

been doing for you. You can start fasting once every three weeks before slowly reducing the time frame as you wish.
- Not one system works the same way for everyone. So choose a plan and use it for your taste.
- You will need to be fully aware of how your body responds to a periodic fasting program. Your body plan will determine what you eat, what time to eat, when to exercise, how many calories, etc. Putting all these things together will ensure that you are in control of the fasting process and, ultimately your weight.
- You don't want to hurry when you see fat flying through your bones. Many of us are impatient and get rid of certain foods one after the other because they don't work fast enough. You need to understand that for health purposes, losing weight should be a slow and slow process. Losing two pounds a week is just okay.
- Take part in your daily activities while you are in a hurry as this is a time-travel method. Being inactive will keep your mind focused on food, and you can guess the result here.

The most important piece of advice is that you do not have to eat all the time. As with health, there is a time for everything we have set for ourselves. So it also applies to your diet. Fasting is not ironclad, work on it, and set up a plan that works for you.

Chapter 5: Successful, Fasting, Eating and Eating

Most people will experience the effect of periodic fasting. They eat well in certain windows and make sure food is healthy when eaten. However, if you want to improve your performance and burn more fat, it is important to add your workout to your daily routine. This chapter outlines the proper training and exercise strategies to take during a quick workout.

In fact, a recent study by the Swedish Institute of Sports and Health Science showed that lowering the total amount of carbohydrates in a diet can cause the body to burn calories more efficiently and increase the capacity for muscle growth. In this study, ten cyclists who received an hour of interval training reached 64% of their maximum aerobic capacity. Glycogen levels are low or normal in their diet or before exercise intervention.

Ten biopsies were performed before the exercise and three hours after the exercise. The results indicate that exercise in glycogen depletion can increase mitochondrial biogenesis. This is the process by which new mitochondria can form within the cell. The authors of this study believe that low glycogen intake may be helpful in improving the oxidative capacity.

Part of the reason for making your current fasting state is that the body has ways to protect and protect your tissues from debris. So, if you naturally use very little energy during fasting, the body will start to break down other tissues, but it will not slow down the active tissue you are using.

Exercise While Maintaining Muscle Mass

Many experts believe that about 80% of the health benefits from a healthy diet come from food. The rest will be from sports. This means that if you want to lose more weight, you need to focus on eating the right foods. However, it is important to note that exercise and diet are necessary.

Investigators learned the details of the 11 participants who participated in the "Big Loser" program. Total body fat for participants, total energy cost, and resting rate were measured three times. At the beginning of the program, the measurement was taken after six weeks and 30 weeks. Using a personalized food model, researchers can calculate the effects of diet and exercise changes on weight loss to understand how everyone achieves this goal.

Researchers have found that diet itself is a major cause of weight loss. However, about 65% of the loss of weight originates from body fat. It happens due to the leaning of muscles. Exercise alone will result in a decrease in fat and a slight increase in the number of soft muscles.

Exercise and Fasting Together

If you want to find a workout program that works out, add high-intensity training, and occasional fasting, you need to combine certain things. When you do this, if you feel that you do not have enough energy to keep up with exercise, it's time to make some changes. Often reducing hours in an empty stomach will make the difference. Fasting indoors can make you feel good. If you can't hurry, it's time to change your strategy.

There are two important points to keep in mind when exercising at regular intervals. The first is about mealtimes. Fasting indoors is not just about limiting calories. You don't have to starve yourself to get the best results. Instead, this is just time to plan meals, so you don't have to eat most of the day. You can eat out of a small window, maybe at night or later in the day. So, if your dinner is limited to between 4 and 7, you will be fasting for 21 hours.

For most people, it is good to fast for 12 to 18 hours. Most people like to fast for 16 hours because it fits their busy schedule. You can find a way that best suits your needs while making sure you get all the benefits.

If you can't completely stop eating during the day, you can limit your dose of small, simple hypoglycemic foods. This includes cooking a pack of boiled eggs, Whey protein, vegetables, and fruits every four to six hours. It doesn't matter what you decide to eat; it is best to avoid eating at least three hours before bedtime. Doing this can help you minimize the damage to your system and can make periodic fasting easier.

In addition, on the day of exercise, you should break the fast by restoring food. On days when you have to exercise while fasting, you need to take a snack of about 30 minutes after your workout. Adding Whey Protein made to a meal can help rejuvenate the body's tissues.

After dinner, it's best to fast and have a great dinner that night. Eat a balanced diet after each workout. This will ensure that your body receives the demand for energy, and no muscle or brain damage. Don't skip these foods and make sure you get them within 30 minutes of your use.

If you think it is difficult to fast for 12 to 18 hours, you can get the same benefits from exercise and fasting by eating breakfast and exercise as soon as you have an empty stomach in the morning. This is because eating a large meal before exercise, especially foods with high carbohydrate content, will hinder the sympathetic nervous system and reduce the effect of fat burning during exercise.

So many people are taught that they need to get more carbohydrates before exercise in order to gain endurance and see results; it goes against your goal. Eating carbohydrates activates the parasympathetic nervous system, which promotes energy storage and stores calories and carbohydrates in the body. If you are exercising and doing quick exercises from time to time, this may be the last thing you want, so it is better to exercise faster to get better results.

Use Your Fitness Tips a Lot

Exercise is not necessarily difficult. Exercise and lots of exercise can help you feel good, build muscle, and lose weight. Other ways to ensure that you do well during regular exercise include:

- Start small - if you've never done a weight-lifting plan before, you need to start slowly. Even if you return to an existing workout, it's important to remember the changes and slow down until you know how they will affect your performance.

- Increase your weight when you feel relaxed - it's important to continue to gain weight when you start to feel comfortable. As time goes by, the weight used to start the work will start to feel easier, and if you don't make any changes, you will find that the results will be slower. This does not mean that you want to force your body to exceed the limit, but rather that if you want to achieve continued success; you need to increase the difficulty of a regular exercise program.

Reduce the Number of Times and Gain Weight Is Best for Soft Muscles - If at All

If you want to build muscle, consider reducing the amount of repetition when you increase your weight. This will get rid of your body faster and give you better results.

Don't forget to warm up and relax - just because you have to change your eating habits and can't give you excuses to slow down the warmth and calm of your daily workout. It takes at least five minutes to stretch the muscles at the beginning and end of the operation, which not only improves athletic performance but also reduces the chances of injury.

Focus on bodybuilding - sometimes paying too much attention to the weight it can lift while exercising. However, having the right form is really important. It is better to exercise properly and lightweight than to gain weight and not do it right.

Chapter 6: Intermittent Fasting Diet.

In the whole chapter, we will look at fat storage inside our bodies and how to burn it.

How This Fat Is Stored and Burnt?

This type of fasting has been looked at as a helpful factor to consider in one's health as it burns fats and eventually makes one lose his weight. How is this tool effective? Before we go in detail on this issue you are supposed to know how your body stores energy it acquires from intakes, how it uses the energy, and the roles played by body hormones in the body functions. In the circle of human life its either you store energy in your body or burn that energy and calories attained by body tissues every day.

This concludes that your body is either using energy (sugar) or storing it inform of fat or glycogen. Whether you are mobile or immobile in your daily chores you have the ability to burn your fats and calories and even sugar that is stored in excess amounts in the body.

According to statistics, mobility does not play many roles in the fat burn process; researchers suggest a 2:3 percentage in the loss equation. Human beings burn fat in many ways even when they are not moving, they will still lose it upon a smart guide discussed in the below chapters. The body of a human being will tend to expend its energy as it does its normal functioning according to BMR and BMR.

Even though the body might be consuming and burning all the calories all the excess is stored for use, and it's the energy stored that makes intermittent fasting a successful deal. As much as your body stores sugar and burns it weight loss is geared by less eating, and more exercises will this book will be your first beat of gearing success in losing weight and maintaining your body healthier. You will see the results at the end, and count fails to get back to normal eating and lifestyle.

What should you do to make it a success in losing weight? To get the image of all these two principals will not only guide you but also be of a great impact if practiced with concern; the principle of storing and burning sugar and how that sugar can be used for energy is your first option. The second principle is the role played by body hormones in the body functions.

How Is Energy Stored in Our Bodies?

The body of a human body can store energy in two ways, either in fat or glycogen. For instance, if you take a yum diet it is broken down into small and simple macronutrients ready to be absorbed in the body bloodstreams and transported in the body tissues for normal body functioning. In these processes, carbohydrates are broken down into glucose that is transmitted in the body cells for energy and with the excess stored as Glycogen through the glycogenesis process. Our bodies are meant for storing energy as fats, which are eventually broken down into energy through a process known as lipolysis, but only when it is in huge amounts is when is stored.

How Is the Stored Energy Used in Body Functioning?

Immediately the body cells require a lot of energy than the one needed (low blood sugar) by the bloodstreams. Glycogen is converted to glucose by the glycogenolysis process. The glycogen stores fats and then get back it after being emptied to digest the available fats by lipolysis process raising blood sugar level to its normality, and the whole process will mean breaking down of fats. To summarize on the process;

- Excess glucose is turned to glycogen and stored once it is activated by a high

  sugar level.
- Once glycogen is filled up the glucose stored in excess is converted to fat and

  stored.
- Blood sugar level drop symbolizes glycogen breakdown to glucose

- Fat is broken down once the glycogen stores are emptied

To this far we have roughly looked on how our bodies function through storing of fats, breaking them down into energy/burning them. Below we will discuss the hormones responsible for controlling these processes.

Hormones

Body hormones are the most associated with one's moods. They play a big role in someone's weight loss. The secretion of hormones is of a great deal with your body as it rises from glands, each with a purpose. For instance, when blood sugar level rises, it plays the role of releasing insulin. Below are the key hormones responsible for weight loss.

Insulin Rising of blood sugar level activates insulin release leading to low blood sugar. This is because insulin helps in the transmission of glucose in the body cells for energy with the excess insulin taken into the liver. This makes the insulin to operate with much ease and start breaking down fats into glycogen. When you eat, your blood sugar level rises to stimulate the production of insulin that is of great importance. High secretion of insulin is activated by huge intakes of carbohydrates and lots of eating which results in the constant intake of sugar in the body. Since the main role of insulin is to store energy constant intake and eating of carbohydrates means that your body is storing a lot of carbohydrates which means that failure to take action to burn it will lead to weight gain and you will be at the risk of getting back to the weight loss procedures.

This is because the insulin will begin to resist its functions and the body will have to resist its functioning which means that more secretion of insulin will have to take place to fight against high sugar levels in the blood which will lead to overload of storing forcing liver to make convert of fats into glucose and start gaining weight through fattening. This is because glucagon is broken down once blood sugar level drops in order to raise blood sugar in the bloodstreams. Glucagon also stimulates adipose tissues that break the fat stores for bloodstreams. You are supposed to know that glucagon does the opposite of insulin in support of body functions. This leads to an energy-burning state which is geared by when insulin releases two hormones, which will be discussed in the chapters below.

Human Growth Hormone (HGM)

The weight loss perspective you need to know is that Human growth Hormones are triggered by enough sleep, low blood sugar level, and enough exercising. Human growth hormone functioning depends on different factors; for example, when children are sleeping their HGM will help their bones to grow but to the same as for adults. In relation to weight loss, the human growth hormone helps to regulate low blood sugar by breaking down the stored fats and growing muscles. Once you are an underweight loss, you are needed to lean on the activity of HGM and its production in your body.

Under endocrinology, the human brain senses insulin-like growth factors in the body and suppresses HGM release in the body and this clarifies the method of diagnosing overproduction of HGH which is done by giving sugary drink to the affected hence promoting drop of the HGH level drop with the meaning that high consumption of carbohydrates and sugary foods will not only go to give you high blood sugar but also overturn the release of HGH. These hormones do not stimulate adipose tissue break down to store fats, which means that it is never in the system with the role of stimulating muscle growth and bone density. This is caused by the release of fat cells, which means that the more fat cells you are having, the more leptin is released in the body to help in stabilizing weight by regulating hunger, appetite, and satiety.

Leptin

Leptin level refers to the number of fats you are having with your body. The more body fat you have, the more leptin you are having in your bloodstreams. The less body fat you are having, the less leptin your bloodstreams will be having, with the aim of losing weight drop-in body fat that leads to a drop-in leptin level resulting in an increase in appetite. With this mechanism in your tips, you will understand the reason why the loss of weight makes someone feel like he/she eat a whole horse if allowed to.

Just Like insulin, the body can develop leptin resistance because when you are overweight, the excess amounts of leptin in the bloodstreams might make the body to build immunity, meaning that even when you carry a lot of fats, the leptin doesn't work well to overwhelm your appetite, which may encourage overeating and cause inequality of the hormones discussed above.

Eating on the intermittent fast is very simple and with very many complications as it is always upon your choice to continue with your eating behaviors or add a new diet and eventually see the end results. The ketogenic diet can better you if allowed to as it helps in limiting your carbs and reducing hunger and eventually burn your fats quickly. While under intermittent fasting there is no need to go on a specific meal as you can rarely get results at the end, in fact, you are supposed to eat healthy food on this diet plan since with this diet plan one is expected to drop his eating habit during the day to not more than eight hours but note that using these time gaps to eat fast foods such as snacks will still drive you into issues for you will not be able to lose your weight once you eat these fast foods as they are rich sources of calories with some other unhealthy foods which will give you a huge intake in every time you have them as food.

Though you might have small intakes of these unhealthy foods, you will stop your entire process of burning fats and fail to increase your weight loss effort. To this far you might have noticed that eating snacks and fast foods will definitely fail your effort of weight loss because they are unhealthy and causes the same problems that you encounter before starting the process.

When you have an unhealthy diet, you will find that you are hungry often and you will struggle with getting through your fasting periods with less comfort because many processed and fast foods contain chemicals and preservatives that are designed to make you hungry often in the event where you intend to start prayer and fasting even if for a whole month it's the high time to start eating healthier food or diets. This does not mean that you are supposed to avoid junk foods and sweets on occasions as it does not have set guidelines for what you are allowed to eat as it simply sets the times that you are allowed to eat. Eating a little snack and junk meal is fine. As long as you have it during your eating windows and only do it on occasions though it may be hard, always eating healthier will provide you with better results.

The trick to making this practice successful is always eating healthier. The first thing that you need to put into consideration is eating plenty of fruits and vegetables or including them in every diet with much majoring on fresh produces as they are best because they provide lots of essential nutrients that your body requires to stay healthy. Consider filing your plate with fruits and vegetables in every meal so that you ensure that you are getting the nutrients that are essential for someone's health. Eating a wide variety of products is very important to ensure that you are getting what your body requires without adding in lots of calories.

Next, you are supposed to go with some good sources of protein. You should consider options like lean ground beef, turkey, and chicken. Having some bacon and other fatty meats on occasion is acceptable, but don't overdo it. Eating a lot of fish will help you get the healthy fatty acids that the body needs to function appropriately.

Healthy sources of dairy help someone to stay lean while giving his body the calcium it needs. You can have some options like milk, yogurt, cheese, sour cream, and many others. Make sure that you monitor the salts and sugars that are not healthy for your body.

You are accepted to have some carbs on such a diet. Carbs have become a bit of a bad reputation because very many diet plans recommend that you avoid them. The most important thing is eating the carbs that are healthy and of benefit to your health. Foods such as snacks, White bread, and pasta are sugar made in disguise and should be avoided. Going with both whole grain and whole wheat options when it comes to your carbs will ensure that you get all the nutrition that you will need. Taking a well-balanced meal will be the key to ensuring that you feel good when you are on an intermittent fast as your body will remain strong as well as healthy at all times. You will be able to mix the meals that you choose, so as to get the best results when you go on this kind of fasting.

You can also have with you a snack and remember how often you are having it because when you are eating junk foods, you will get disappointed when you go to measure your weight to the scale as you will find that you are adding your weight instead of losing it. You can have as many pleasures on occasions as well as many junk meals, but make sure that it is not exceeded in your diets.

Using the Ketogenic Diet with Intermittent Fasting

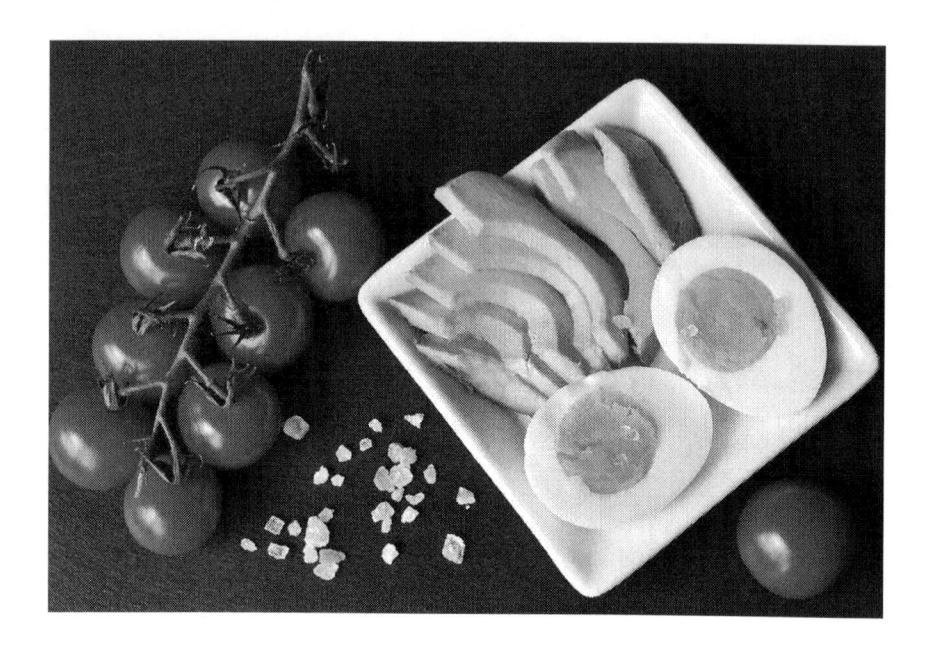

Many people choose to go for a ketogenic diet while doing an intermittent fast to help them remain healthy. The ketogenic diet includes high fat, moderate proteins, and low carb diets that help someone to burn fat quickly while reducing his dependency on sugary meals. There is a lot to love with this diet plan because when combined with the intermittent fasting, someone is sure to get great results in no time.

It's possible to use both of these diet plans together. Intermittent fasting is focused on the times of day when you will eat, and the ketogenic diet on what to eat during those periods. For someone who would like to balance his blood sugar level and want to lose weight more efficiently, combining these two diet plans together will be very effective.

For intermittent fasting, you should limit the hours that you can eat. Instead of spreading your meals and snacks throughout the day, you should limit it to just a few hours. Most people choose to only eat between ten and six and fit their macronutrients into that time. Others will take two or three days during the week where they are not allowed to eat and fit their nutrients into the other days of the week.

The point is, you are limiting the amount of time that you eat, forcing you to think about the foods you consume. You also get the benefit of more fat burning and weight loss, when practicing intermittent fasting.

During the times when you are allowed to eat, you will need to stick to the macronutrients that we have learned above that are approved for the ketogenic diet. You will still remain with high fat and moderate protein plan even while on intermittent fasting. You will be required to be more cautious about the times you eat the major nutrients though you can still follow the ketogenic diet plan.

If you want to get these benefits of intermittent fasting or you want to increase your weight loss efforts, then adding this diet in with the ketogenic diet is the most effective. You can test with different types of intermittent fasting options that are available and see which one fits into your schedule for the best of you. Of course, if you find the ketogenic diet effective or intermittent fasting very difficult, you can at all times stick with the ketogenic diet and not fast and still see good results.

It is very vital to recall that you don't have to follow the ketogenic diet plan if you are on an intermittent fast. Many people go choose other healthy diets instead of choosing to go on the ketogenic diet. Though, there are many people who will choose to go with the ketogenic diet along with intermittent fasting because it is very easy to follow, and it allows one to lose more fat.

Eating on the intermittent fast does not have to be difficult for you. You can opt to pick out the foods that you want to eat, although it is important to go with food that is fresh and whole, and that will fill you to burn your fat and help you see yourself losing weight.

Chapter 7: Tips to Help You Succeed in Intermittent Fasting

In order to ponder the number of intervals to fast, it will be more viable if one has to choose a style that befits him well. There are different approaches to follow. It could be 12:7 method, or 10:4. The first one is fasting for twelve hours that is, through the better part of the day (even during the sleeping hours), then eight hours to eat food. Then 10:4 methods it entails ten-hour fast followed by a four-hour eating window. Both of these provisions a person can opt to choose when to start even as one pleases. You can cease your fast at noon and consume food at seven in the evening.

Moreover, if the breakfast is more important to you, you can opt to partake late-day snacks then eleven to six evening window to which could prove better for you. Another person could prefer a long span of fasting. This could be composed of 4:2 approaches; this constitutes consuming food for four days in a week and taking the two days as fasting days. The amazing thing about this dieting is that it be customized for someone to choose what he finds appealing or get the same sort of results.

Some of these alternatives could be: having easy swaps of options will make one not run out of order cooks. The positive side of intermittent fasting is its simplicity. Do not resort to unnecessary ways of cooking your own food from the rest of the family meals. For instance, one can make a dish of pasta mixed with Bolognese stew for an evening meal, or spaghetti noodles, for the group and stewed noodles for him. Or offer a plate of lukewarm tortillas and heartwarming lettuce for wraps. These sorts of swaps can take a very small amount of time to prepare. There will be times when interval fasting will be daunting to adapt because someone will have to change some dieting patterns, but the efficacy can come in many ways. Then, in the long run, it can be easier to enhance your energy, lose weight gains, curb against diabetic maladies, cancer, and junk foods.

The intermittent fasting is best than other alternatives out there, but it needs a lot of effort. Some of the things one can bear in mind are: gulping a lot of water which can make one hydrated, and belly become a bit fuller; otherwise, the stomach will always be tormenting due to hunger pangs. Drinking tea and coffee will suppress hunger and unwanted appetites. But do not take caffeinated drinks when about to sleep because that will make one unable to doze. Make your mode of life to be hectic, the reason being that on an empty stomach one can be less active. If you are busy you can attain a lot, avoid hunger, and avoid long periods of hunger spells that appear like long periods of years. Please do not be hard on yourself. When it comes to new eating habits you can make your days filled with many activities. You should be flexible because intermittent fasting comes with its downsides. You do not have to go with the crowd. Mixing and matching the schedule that works is good. Remember, intermittent fasting is about having the self-will to do as one pleases.

Then a person could try to make it a monthly trial. Meaning the probationary period could be from three weeks to four weeks. If someone is not adapting well, it means that there is not ample time to make adjustments. So a certain amount of time is needed to check out whether it works or not. Additionally, one can opt to experiment with alternative fasting methods. What could be feasible to a particular person might be not workable to another person. If you discern that one type of fasting ids better and more applicable than the other application that fits you. The point is that the experiment is all that is needed to make a solid conclusion. Then a person can commence by delaying and denying himself breakfast drastically. Pushing a breakfast in a gradual process every week or so, then you can come into terms with intermittent fasting without too much ado.

For example, if you usually take food at nine o'clock morning you can wait up till ten o'clock and then consume your week's breakfast. Then you can move on taking the same breakfast to ten o'clock. Then you can continue shifting the eating patterns up to midday.

During the start of morning hours, taking a few cupsful of water will be okay. Remember that the reason you feel so hungry in the morning hints that you took nothing as food. So the first thing is to get a glass of water as someone wakes up. Then if there is a need for gaining weight and toning up, it makes sense to it would be wise to resort to weight exercises as a routine. While it will not be wise to start too many things, especially when someone is on a startup route, but as soon as the body adapts to the fasting style, there is a need to move things up. Then there will always be surprises because the body can sustain itself despite too much intensity and many hindrances along the path of improvement.

Intermittent fasting every person has to live up at a time. It can be fascinating as long as there is a balance in the long run.

The typical diet is all about the 'forbidden foods,' but the intermittent fasting means that you cannot preplan your meals. Meaning there is no way to turn around the hours, so long as there is no constancy. Consequently, there is no way someone cannot involve himself, as far as a delicious and a fake dessert does not end up into nine to eight.

Recall being around all nice smelling foods; there is a heavy temptation to get a bite. So make it a policy to get out of the house. If you have kids who needed your attention, exert yourself in an activity that keeps your mindset occupied?

There is a need to take more protein foods and healthy fats because sufficient protein in every meal makes an individual have a controllable appetite and aid in buttressing muscles with energy.

An excellent amount of fats to more energy and a long span of a full belly. We can give credit to many dieticians for giving us many advises on our meals, but sometimes we need to try best to check what works for us or not. The majority of people consume too many carbohydrates and take other unbalanced portions. But the problems can be rectified by taking into consideration the macros of the foods we take. Additionally, when you are taking your favorite delicacy make it a deal that you fill your plate to the brim so that the next window would be easy as possible.

Avoid the worst of all junk foods most of the times people can resort to non-bodybuilding foods but always make it a resolve to have a balanced diet so that you provide your body with sufficient nutrition even if you are about to fast.so it is essential to note that a huge part of intermittent fasting is to gain the amount calories which has been snapped up during the eventual part of the week-long fasting.

If you drench up your body with high– calorie junk when you are embarking on an eating window what could be the consequence is, your hard work is being undone. Recall making decisive options entirely will finally enhance the overall effectiveness of your weight harm efforts, assured.

This journal could prove to be gigantic and important because it can make you keep track of everything from the outset. Someone can use modern gadgets if there he finds that more viable, but some old-fashioned folks using a journal proves easier.

Ideally, it can help also to count the number of no-fasting hours, mood swings at that moment, both positive and negative. This way you can monitor the progress. If there are fits of anger let us say on Tuesday the reason could be that the body is coming into grips with the new fasting you have been up to or that a certain diner you took is still being channeled to your system.it is so hard to discern if there are patterns of loss gains, or moving on the right track healthy lifestyle if you do not document. The best thing is to take a picture of oneself or look yourself in a mirror so as to have something to meditate on later or maybe survey progress

Ride out the Hunger Waves

Pangs of hunger do not endure for a long time, but they can be harrowing. But the moment they emerge, they can be intolerable so you can resort to huger waves. Opposite of the popular opinion that when hunger comes up, it eats up you inside more and more till you sense death, but it subsides depending on the way you can make it through. When someone is hungry what happens to their body is hydration. a particular body may exhibit dehydration by having symptoms of hunger when what needs to be done is just take a cup of water.

Start Gradually

When embarking on a new lifestyle or grappling with intermittent fasting the food advice is to do it gradually. Everybody needs time to adapt and transition itself without haste. For instance, if you are fasting through the normal dinner time until six in the morning make sure you see yourself through without any food around even the ensuing day even stretching up to lunchtime. Some folks have the inclination to get into anything new without any forethought, and they push themselves through the hard spans of times and cravings. But the best of all conveniences gradual process is the best way to travel no matter how rocky it is. In conclusion, we can draw a lot from intermittent fasting; also, we should not have unfounded expectations from weight loss, good body posture no matter how strict the fasting path might be.

Meanwhile, there will be jiffies of weight loss, as the body's systems funnel itself to the trials. But everything will most likely totally change eventually after the fasting period. This can be visible during the initial weeks of transition as the body will be trying cling on to everything that to the time it figures itself out. But the time it figures the process, later on, everything will come to join the dotted path to follow through. Every diet is meant to have weight gains or loss paradigm. This could be part of weight gain or loss, and it cannot be controlled. But there are consistent and feasible measures that will prove adaptable and workable, but the futile thing is to try to change things up whimsically because this can spiral into a more problematic conundrum of events. Whereas if you pursue a positive course and exert oneself to the good work, the fine results will be eminent and visible before you come to realize.

Always bear in mind any strenuous physical activity requires precautions in the same case our intermittent fasting needs lot care because our very souls are involved and depend on it. The health benefits cannot be underestimated because it can prevent diseases and enhance spiritual wellbeing. Even those who are overweight can help to cut down the body mass as well. There are those with eating disorders, so they should not strenuously exert themselves on it. So in hindsight, timing your meals can improve your wellbeing, control weight, and most of all, make you physically active. So the resolve to achieve better results is good regardless of distractions one has to encounter along the way, but the payback will be worth pursuing.

Chapter 8: Most FAQ(s) on Intermitted Fasting

There are simple questions that need to arise from your mind about intermittent fasting. We will be discussing these questions very clearly. What is it needed for intermittent fasting is to enjoy the best out of it to be a simple practice and be of help to you?

Who Should Fast and Not?

This type of fasting is meant for everyone who wishes to reduce his/her fat and the willingness to make it a success in losing weight. As we discussed earlier, it is meant for reducing calories by paving a focus on healthy eating. This reflects that you are not supposed to get into this plan if you need special nutrients in your body due to its characteristic of less food consumption. For instance, if you are pregnant, breastfeeding, and underweight, this diet plan should not concern you at all; otherwise, you should ask for a recommendation from your doctor.

Group two type of people who should not attempt this diet plan are those suffering from Diabetes either type 1 or type 2 and high uric acid they are supposed to take the caution of seeking doctors' advice.

Can Someone Starve While Fasting?

It is a misconception that you can starve while fasting as long as you are healthy fit as intermitted fasting is an effective tool in reducing fats stored in the body and burning them for energy during the starving days. When it comes to fasting, it is all about your wellness, some opinions posted by people against fasting myths are that fasting makes one starve, lose muscles, feel hungry and start overeating after undergoing fasting. As we discussed earlier this is false as all these myths make one lose weight, burn fats, and overcome unnecessary fatness. For instance, if you are struggling with being overweight this is the right book for your weight loss. The myth of starving, which is the most common, is greatly reasoned out by the eating that someone does in a whole year and the intake of calories in those diets with losing one whole week without food. No starving that can be evident in this fasting its benefit and benefit. Just try it and thank yourself later! The body of a human being can stay for even two weeks without food, and you are seen walking very comfortably and without anybody noticing whether you are fasting.

What Side Effects Do They Come with Fasting?

Several effects will come after you are done with your fasting. The effects that someone encounters with this type of fasting are very manageable if you wish to start. After getting back to normal when you are done with burning the stored fats in the body. For example, lack of roughage in the body processes will cause constipation, and since you have gone without food for time this comes as the first side effect. To do away with it you just need some purges to help you in improving your discomfort. The problem of stomach babbling is solved by drinking salty water whereas the problem of headaches that comes often in the first days of fasting is done away by eating salts every morning. You might come across other side effects such as heartburn and dizziness, but after resuming to normal the same you never have the feels at all.

How to Manage the Hunger

The hunger experienced during this time should not worry you as it will pass as it comes. Researchers say that hunger come in waves just like moving water to avoid this hunger while fasting you are supposed to take a soft drink immediately, and you will have no instance of claiming hunger you can also opt to take a cup of tea or coffee and forget about the waves though it will be experienced I the first and second day of fasting. With the third and fourth days, it will be normal to continue the rest of the days you feel of extending your fast. You will manage this because the body has fats that are digested to be a form of energy in the whole fast. Once the hunger pain waves are gone within the second day with the other days it is very cheap and easy for managing the fast. It is very important to have in mind that this is very manageable though for beginners it's a big deal in the first two days due to the habit of the body getting food all through. There two types of fasting 16:8 and 5:2. Practicing either of them is a true indication that you are making yourself strong and even preparing for a life of comfort without obese and free mobility. To prepare for this make sure that you take a balanced meal with every meal as it will make your body to remain strong always and ready. To be in the ability to make this manageable, also you don't leave behind caffeine in your meals because it is a good way to reduce hunger pains when they come in waves. During this type of fast ensure that you keep yourself busy all through to put your mind on the focus of what you are aiming at. If you are already committed to an exercise plan, then you are supposed to ensure that you exercise with much commitment before you break your fats so that your body can get the fuel it needs to make the most of your efforts.

Can Fasting Burn Muscle?

This is a misconception that dwells in almost everyone who fears to fast. This is a myth because, during the fasting periods, the body breaks down the glycogen into glucose to be used for energy purposes, and after the glucose is all gone, the body increases the fat it's breaking down and uses that for energy. Excess amino acids, which build up in the system proteins, can also be used for energy. Fasting is a practice that has been done effectively for a long time. It's safe and effective, and unless you go for weeks without eating there isn't a reason for worrying about losing excess muscles.

 How do I break the fast? Once you are about to break the fast prepare a dish a minute before it is over. A pot of oatmeal is not a good choice; instead, choose an Omelet because it is healthy and has many nutrients. As the end of this fasting is not very nice as it puts one in the point of sustaining in the long moments.

Once you break your fast it is important to do away with moderation for multiple reasons. DO NOT OVER EAT!!! Eat a little dish to withstand a long period you stayed without food, do not also overwork until you resume to normal as the body tissues will have used the stored energy in the tissues.

Can Women Fast?

Women can fast with some exemption, such as if they are underweight, pregnant, or breastfeeding. This is because they require those extra nutrients and should not go so long without eating in intermittent fasting. Otherwise, it is perfect for women to fast as they have huge fats compared to men. Besides, the average weight loss with fasting is the same for men and women, and it is effective for both genders. Though starting intermittent fasting is a challenge for a beginner we are going to discuss tips that will enable you to fast effectively.

Drink a lot of water and prefer water rich in minerals and remain busy in your chores during fasting Drink coffee or tea as they are rich sources of caffeine to suppress your hunger
Find out a support group or a team to help you ride out the hunger waves
Try to go on a low-carb diet because it will help you to reduce your hunger and make your fasting as easy as possible.
Break a fast gently and avoid too much eating in the first days until you get used to normal.

Bonus Tips to Help in Maintaining the Proper Weight

Use of Spices

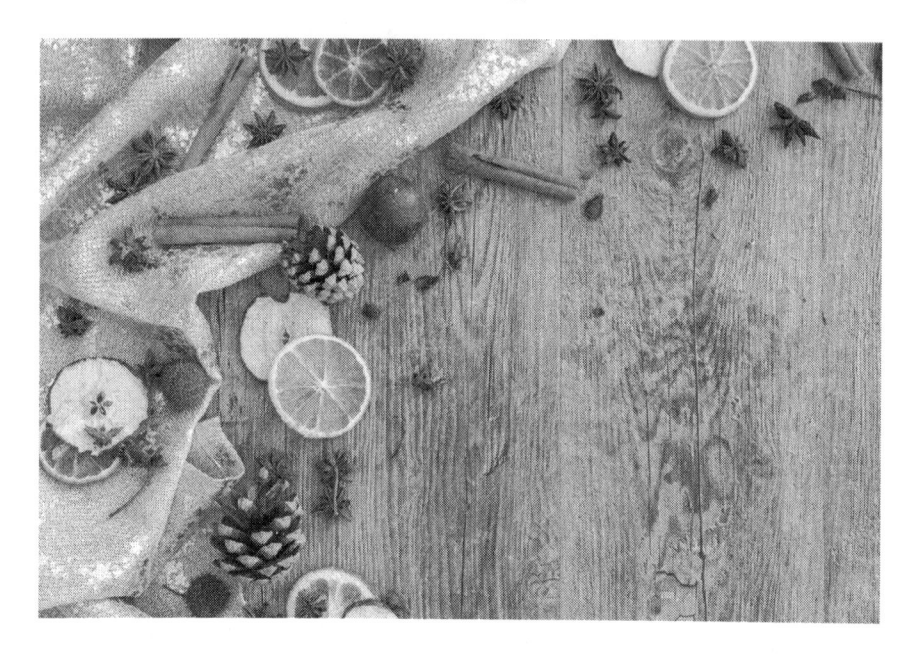

Spices have performed a number of functions ranging from flavor to medicinal purposes since the beginning of humankind. Archaeological studies have found spices from the ruins around the Nile District since 2800 BC. The various types of spices and herbs not only delight our scents, but they also work to preserve human bodies. Countries in the medieval period carried herbs and spices to great heights and used them for purposes ranging from funeral ceremonies, royal ceremonies, and treatments.

In these modern times, we have associated the spices most with the taste qualities they offer to our dishes. Going back to studying the ancient uses of these spices has begun to open a new vista to their potential as a coolant and protect against the powerful antioxidants of fat burning. According to one recent study, the American Journal of Clinical Nutrition reported that adding rich spices to polyphenol in a meat dish reduced the production of Malondialdehyde, which is a product of peroxidation of lipids and is thought to cause cancer. Other studies have confirmed the effectiveness of spices and herbs by using its antioxidant power to fight off harmful substances in our daily diet. For example, do you know that the meat and other products that you produce and like so contain carcinogens?

This, however, can be reduced to a minimum by the addition of spices that prevent the formation of computer-generated cancer. Heterocyclic amine complements are made up mainly of meat, poultry, and seafood that are cooked at high temperatures, especially over fire or frying. We can almost certainly avoid such an important part of our diet, so what do we need to do to reduce the risk associated with consuming such products? Just introduce spices and herbs to brighten up the flavor of your barbecue and products at the same time for you and your loved ones. Common ingredients such as cumin, turmeric, and dozens of others are helpful in reducing HCA production. Spices and herbs not only reduce your risk of cancer but also serve as a barrier and cure against many other diseases from diabetes to common colds.

A 2011 study revealed that cinnamon and cloves because of its high hypolipidemic properties reduced blood cholesterol by approximately 65% in subjects during the study period. How do you explain weight loss in a high-fat diet during reading? This is the effect of the spices added to the diet of the articles during the frame.

As you continue to experience the wonderful potential of herbs, it is important to increase your use of these anti-inflammatory drugs. You can combine the following steps along the way to good health;

Take herbs and herbs with standard health supplements and not for the extra benefit they can give you. It is appropriate to eat foods that are rich in antioxidants, e.g., Spices, herbs, vegetables, fresh fruits, etc. To make your meal a great experience. As long as studies are ongoing regarding a particular disease inhibition of spice skills, that should not stop you from taking antioxidant-rich foods. We know for sure that spices contain significant amounts of antioxidants, but the lack of information lies in how this relates to good health and the benefits it provides us that we use regularly.

Don't limit yourself to specific spice and herbs; check the entire rainbow light. By trying a little of this and adding some of that to your diet, you will be getting the best of the delicious and healthy ingredients they have.

You should take your spices and herbs in any way you can. If you find a garden, then it makes perfect sense that you can use many new spices. However, if you can get your hands on some new herbs, dried ones will do the job correctly and often and over new treatments. The UCLA School of Medicine's research into herbs and spices found that they keep their essentials even though they are dry.

Details of the specific health benefits can be substantially better compared to sugar, fat, and salt. Spices bring out the subtle flavor, aromas, and flavor of your dishes and are healthy for your body. If you are on a diet or are looking for ways to get rid of those stubborn body fats, spices can come in to replace sugar and other artificial particles. We are so attached to the traditional ways of satisfying our languages and not paying enough attention to our bodies that the most common spices available may not have been recognized. Cinnamon is a great place for sugar in your tea, coffee, cereals. Your taste buds may be at war with you at first, but gradually the taste you get becomes more normal as your body begins to experience the great health benefits associated with its use.

There are many ways that when combined can be of effective remedies to keep your health in good condition all the year. They are relatively cheap with the process of making them so simple that even a young child can put them together. So getting into the crust of the remedies, there are few spices that you can implement into your daily meal plans for a healthy life. With this, I will be putting out a few powerful spices that work with much ease and that you might take and mix with any menu you might choose to come up with.

As much as you take all these measures to be cautious, especially if you have any severe ailments and undergoing treatment with medications, you are supposed to get in touch with a general consultant before you consume any spice or herb.

Cinnamon

This is the spice that lowers someone's blood sugar because it possesses an aroma that is quite lovely. If you might be dealing with diabetes, either type 1 or type 2, this is one spice that should adorn in your kitchen cabinet all the time. This is because constant use of this spice gradually pulls you away from the grip of sugar, and makes your body to stop craving for the sweet things. The good thing with this spice is that you get great sweetness without the ability to have harmful effects due to lots of sugar in your system.

This can elevate your risks of coming down with complications associated with diabetes to avoid it add a sprinkle to your tea or coffee or a teaspoon to your juice or any of your favorite drink.

Ginger

This is a light-yellow rhizome that has a sharp and hot taste. It has anti-microbial and anti-inflammatory properties. The fat-burning qualities of ginger are supposed to be marveled at. It is considered to be a digestive fire that paves the way for someone's body to produce digestive enzymes that quickly breaks down nutrients. Moreover, it is an essential spice for the treatment of a lot of your everyday illnesses that you will typically take synthetic and potentially harmful substances into your body to cure. This spice takes care of body pains, common cold, aching of the joints, nausea, and a boatload of other sicknesses. Once taken regularly and on a daily basis either in the form of tea or incorporated into other meals, it serves as a very powerful agent in the reduction of high cholesterol levels in your body. This is a spice that costs someone next to nothing and is ideally suited for a lot of body types without any side effects that are associated with artificial chemical substances someone consumes.

It is one of the best ingredients in improving someone's poor digestion. To get your gastrointestinal system activated daily, you are supposed to ensure that you take a teaspoon of dried ginger powder with warm water and some honey and ensure that it is the first thing you do in the morn at least thirty minutes before having your breakfast. You may also take it in between meals during the day. You can choose to add ginger can to your meals in the fresh form to boil your beef and also sprinkle onto your food to give a boost in your digestion.

With this spice, it not only work on your internal organs but also serves the role of supplying the body's external needs with a soothing and efficient circulation of blood at the surface of the skin. For someone with sore muscles or joints, he/she can make a poultice by adding two teaspoons of dried ginger powder a cup of warm water and gently stir up until there is the formation of a fine paste. Apply it to the spot and massage it into your muscles and start enjoying a soothing relief. It is very relevant to ensure that this mixture does not come in contact with your nose or eye, and to perfect it you are required to ensure that you wash your hands properly after handling ginger because of its fiery nature.

Onion and Garlic

Both of these spices are excellent cholesterol-lowering abilities, but most folks stay away from them because of the pungent odor associated with them, especially garlic. They have been used for quite a long time for their medicinal properties and for spicing foods. Onion and garlic stimulate the production of digestive enzymes, which breaks down fatty acid deposits. Garlic has a broader spectrum of action compared to the onion, and its active ingredients are stronger than those found in onions. They are useful in the cleansing of the liver, lowering high blood pressure, bacterial infections and they are not limited to gastrointestinal disorders and the common cold.

So now let's get into the act of using these new spices effectively. You can start by grinding on cloves of garlic and onions by dicing them up and adding some vinegar and manage to make a zingy salad without forgetting a dash of honey that might add some much-needed mellow taste to the mixture. This is convenient in the treatment of respiratory tract problems. I expect that you know onions and garlic are used for cooking in boiling, steaming, or frying specific foods. The healing effect of these two great spices on our bodies cannot be over-estimated.

If you wish onions and garlic can be consumed in powder or oil forms this comes down to suit you at any given point of time. You may choose to dissolve the powder in warm water and drink or take a clove or two of garlic two to three times every day; all of this will depend on your choice. It is important to note that if you have issues with one's gallbladder, take a full berth around garlic and onions and keep walking once you taste them, you are going to have severe pains for quite a long time.

Turmeric

This plant has been referred to as the "Top Dog of Spices." It helps the breakdown of food down the system, purifies the liver, and getting rid of poisonous substances from the human body.

So there is no need to take an anti-inflammatory prescription that can have detrimental effects on you, but turmeric can go well with your body.

It can ease off stress, cure diabetic problems, remedy digestive problems, control the diabetic impacts, and the endless cases of diseases. It has an unmatchable capability to preserve foods. Due to its potential to prevent the virus, it has been verified to give a blow to cancer-causing pathogens. There are no documented cases of people being affected by the overconsumption of turmeric. Any person can take the ground form of turmeric with tea, or coffee even incorporating it with other meals. The importance of this kind of spice is that it breaks down the buildup of fats inside the tissues. The incessant use of turmeric can make and steer up the digestive system and the body's membrane be4coming glossy.

Those who have been taking ginger and turmeric, especially for a long time when they were craving alcohol as the addictive vice to them reported more mental tranquility and superficial improvement of overall confidence. Then a little wonder is that they sensed less craving to smoke and consume alcohol. Some other additional advantages of the same spices are minimized acne and other skin blemishes that ensue from sweating and hormones. The blistering creamy sparkle of this amazing spice gives someone an aura of mellowness to his coffee as breakfast. At the best of all times, this wonderful spice does not end any breakfast delicacy, but it is part and parcel of those who comprehend its usefulness. So in essence, everyone should be a darling of this first-rate spice and experience the advantages that stream out of it.

Cayenne Pepper

This is also a very piquant and hot spice. The very hotness results from the capsaicin which is ever-present in hot peppers from chili to jalapenos. Due to the existence of the active components in the peppers, you can get the identical paybacks from all of these spices. Its principal purpose is to give a new lease of life to our metabolism, almost double our normal functionality when we have any food devoid it. After a plateful of jalapeno spiced food like barbecue, pizza someone feels re-ignition of metabolism, and the heart pace becomes stabilized. This is a fulfilling way to limit your eating longings as you get jam-packed quickly while your metabolism upsurges at the same time. So this is one ordinate spice that can aid in the dropping of excess body weight in a fine way.

Chances are that we have some other fascinating recipes that can bring a smile to our hearts mostly when we wake up in the morning. The day becomes lightened – so trying up cayenne pepper and lemons is the best alternative. It gets you straight out of bed, lights up your day when you put it in your breakfast. So it is good to try cayenne pepper and squash of lemon. Simply squeeze the lemon juice into the jar or any apparatus and give it a sprinkle of the aforementioned pepper in it. It can provide a jolt of excellent feeling in your system.

Black Pepper

This an important herb for strengthening one's gastrointestinal glares, arousing appetite, and more so cleansing organs.
It also helps in more production of hydrochloric acid, which makes the digestive system more viable. It curtails common diseases like common cold, fevers, and allergens. There are some other acute ailments like anorexia, liver diseases, nervous breakdowns; all those can be cured by administering black pepper. As a fact just take two spoonsful of black pepper, lace-up it with some honey, and maintain that daily as healthy takings.

Cumin

Incredibly, this spice has been confirmed in many areas of study to burn Belly fats three times than any other confirmed methods. Mainly take a small amount of water or mix it with morning tea daily and keep surveillance of fats around the waist being erased out. This is just one incredible spice that has been showed in studies to burn belly fat three times faster healthier than any known method. Just a pinch of warm water or your tea two to three times daily and watch that spare tire around your waist deflate in no time.

Eating Spicy Foods

Tea of Different Flavors

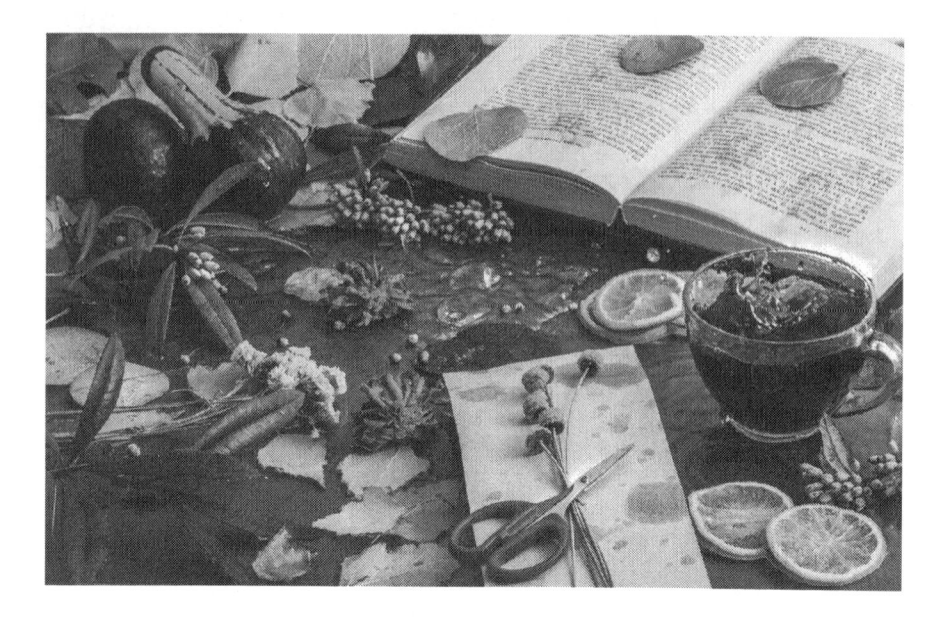

There is this health and vitality that a cup of well-prepared tea rich in antioxidants and earthy flavor can give your day. Entering into your comfort wander around in the evening with a book in hand or just be ready to break through that door to catch the train in the morning. Your cup of tea should give you the kind of comfort you won't get when your fingers are taken, and it should hold you back from accepting that you are not going anywhere else. Building your relationship with this beverage cup brings out some of the benefits of photo-free photography. A cup of tea can be as a standalone drink or eaten after a meal will help your food enter your stomach properly and help your digestion

I will give you a recipe for tea that you would love for life and pass it on to your kids. Now let's get into it. All you need for this recipe is some cinnamon, ginger, and honey. That's all. Surprised? Keep it simple and watch the magic as it unfolds in your body.

Find medium-sized ginger, wash, and peel it. Add it to the kettle and re-add one small cinnamon stick. Pour about 3 cups of water into the mixture and allow boiling for about 25 minutes. You can do more by increasing the number of ingredients if you have more tea lovers around you. You can also store in your refrigerator anytime you need a quick dose of life-giving elixir. So while this mixture is bubbling and the aroma from cinnamon stick fills every corner of your home, your body can't help but wait for the burning fluid that will bring much-needed relief from the forced fay.

After this mixture should boil for a few minutes, dip the liquid into the cavity. You can add honey if you need to soften it a bit, but it is not necessary since the cinnamon has a slightly sweet taste. The flavor explosion that mimics your taste buds is not the same thing you have ever had. It can be taken at any time of the day for your meals or alone.

Herbal Water

Do I need to continue the benefits that water has for life? I don't guess. However, drinking the recommended eight glasses of clean, dirty water can be a major challenge for many of us. Pure water is colorless, odorless, and tasteless. So how is it that we get around to just drinking "normal water" all day for the rest of our lives? We are merely enriching ourselves and stop living a tiring life. To start living a life full of fun with water to use with spices and spices. Get a mug and fill it with eight glasses of water, add three teaspoons of ginger to its wonderful digestive properties, and two slices of cucumber. Find the center lemon, close it, and place it in half. A few freshly squeezed mints leaves give a refreshing taste to the mix and also reduce your hunger pangs and reduce your sugar cravings.

Reduce Salt and Sugar Intake

Spices are great for giving us a taste of junk food and are important in helping us reduce the amount of sugar, salt, and other unwanted foods in our diet. Here are some of the easiest to follow tips for cutting out such food items.

To reduce the salt you use, use less spicy spices, e.g., ginger, onion, garlic, basil, curry, etc. It is also worth checking the labeled spices to make sure no sodium or some form of salt is added to the spice.

To keep your tongue happy, stick with "delicious" spices like cinnamon, nutmeg, allspice, Cardamom, etc. Gradually adding such spices to your daily drinks will see you become healthier as your tongue adapts to changes.

Rules to Consider

When cooking with spices or mustard, always make sure the recipe is well documented. However, when compiling a menu yourself, the amount and type of spice you add to any particular dish depends on your taste buds, and the occasion. Have you ever been in a jam about how to get a recipe that requires fresh spices and herbs but all you have is a dry compliment? Here's an easy way to get an equal amount of fresh spices

½ teaspoon dry ground herbs ¼ teaspoon dried herbs ¼ teaspoon freshly pulled

How many spices and herbs should you put in a bowl if you don't know how to do it? Follow these simple steps, and your diet will go well.

When cooking over a specified amount of people in a recipe, do not assume that it will double the amount of spices you should use. Increase the simple number of ingredients by ½ and taste it and decide when more is needed.

When hot peppers such as chili, jalapenos, cayenne, or red peppers are important ingredients in a bowl, add them slowly in small amounts because the taste becomes stronger as the cooking progresses.

Start any meal by adding ¼ of the necessary spices and adding it as slowly as possible.

The timing of adding spices to any meal is important, and it is also determined by the type of dish you prepare. When adding fresh spices meal, it will come to an end when your cooking is almost done because excessive heat can lead to a loss of flavor. Some very fragrant spices can be sprinkled with food just before it is served or as soon as the food leaves the fire. On the other hand, really heavy spices can last 10 to 15 minutes before a meal is finally ready.

Dried spices are best used in dishes that will be cooked for a long time, and emit their aroma slightly compared to fresh spices.

It is also important to keep your spices and herbs in order to maintain their quality for a very long time. To ensure you get the best out of your spices, store them in dark containers and perhaps on the shelves of your kitchen. Avoid areas where humidity and temperature can occur. Make sure you keep it in air conditioners. When cooking, use dry spoons to take the quantity you need and do not pour your spices into the cooking pot to prevent the smoke from draining and ultimately damage your spices.

No matter how well you store your spice, like any food, it has a shelf life. So your used spices in powdered form, keep for 15 months and unrefined spices, for almost 30 months. To make sure that you do not eventually allow your spices to dissolve, buy small items first until you find out how long it takes to complete them.

Invalid Weight Loss Method

There is no doubt that there are many exercise programs and diet modes that allow you to achieve maximum weight loss with minimal effort, but it is certain that some of these techniques are ineffective, and even if they work, side effects can be harmful to your health. Therefore, you need to be very careful and consult your general practitioner before starting any weight loss program. You need to pay special attention to eating habits, especially when the weight is related to the disease. To avoid wasting time and money to solve things that might not ultimately work for you, here are some things that might not work for your weight loss, as well as suggested long-term alternatives.

Fat-Free and Sugar-Free

Regardless of the harmful effects of excess body fat, fat intake is not completely unhealthy. In fact, fat is one of the food nutrients necessary for the body to stay healthy. On the other hand, you may avoid avoiding sugar while avoiding exposure to fat, or avoiding fat that exposes you to more sugar. In fact, sugar-free products may contain artificial sweeteners, which will also help to gain weight. Even sugar-free drinks contain substances that enhance the taste, which in turn may lead to more sugar exposure. Synthetic fat-free or sugar-free products are not effective. Because you consume more chemicals than sugar or fat, you often eat unhealthily. Instead, stick to natural organic products to lose weight and promote health.

Loading Protein

We all made the wrong idea that too much protein would reduce the rate of eating and, thus the fat content. In fact, eating only protein food means you are depriving the body of other essential nutrients such as fats and carbohydrates. Whether you need to lose weight or not, you need a balanced diet to stay healthy and maintain optimal weight. No nutrient is good for you. You can't just focus on one type of food. You need to balance to get the power you need to lose weight.

Counting Calories

Do you think that the higher the calorie level consumed, the higher the fat achieved? If so, then you have been thinking about all the mistakes. Good nutrition doesn't always mean reducing all calories and avoiding intake. Knowing that not all calories are the same, the calorie quality that enters your body can affect your existing calories, which may surprise you. Similarly, the time of calorie intake can also affect body function. Some calories

Foods from different fruit types or foods have different effects on your body because they cause a mixed reaction in the body. You need to understand the difference between empty calories and good calories. Sticking to healthy foods is the best option when ingesting quality calories, and you don't need to control or calculate calories.

Keep Away from Snacks

Staying away from snacks does not mean completely reducing snacks. Avoid uncontrolled snacks that keep you healthy and away from unnecessary diets, but you need to control the condition of the snacks, and you'll be fine. Just like any addiction, eating less addicted food is better than a diet that completely reduces addiction today and a diet that you don't want to eat snacks tomorrow. Have a healthy nutritious meal, please stick to it, and you don't have to work hard to avoid being bitten in order to lose weight.

Low-Calorie Diet

Although in the history of weight loss programs and diets, most of them are foods with low or controlled calories. If you can't control your body to fit a particular type of diet without having to relapse or turn to junk food or other unhealthy foods, then dieting is useless. These diets often starve and reduce metabolism. Problem will

Once you start your regular diet and have a reasonable calorie in your diet, stop eating. The wise choice is to choose only foods that are commensurate with your physical needs and health requirements.

Get Rid of Dairy Products

Why do most dieters blacklist all dairy products, including ice cream, cheese, and milk? The body also needs milk, and the body needs a lot of milk. In fact, when enough calcium is supplied to the body, the body burns fat at a high rate. Lack of calcium can lead to fat production, allowing you to gain weight while losing weight. Even if it is a low-fat food, be sure to include dairy products in the shopping.

Detoxification

Detoxification is an extreme measure designed to remove toxins from the body, especially the liver. Detoxification products are designed to keep the colon clean, but according to experts, all of these products are nonsense. Your kidneys and liver are doing all the necessary cleaning work. These detox diets are juices that may contain sugar and may not be suitable for your weight level.

Skip Breakfast

Every enlightened person knows that breakfast is something you should not skip because it is crucial. You can't just eat breakfast just because you need to lose weight. Eating light food in the morning is much better than eating it completely because once you don't eat breakfast, you may eat more in the afternoon, which may eventually lead to overeating and also lead to eating food, which will increase your fat level. The more important part of the lunch and the desire to eat again before dinner are all the consequences of skipping breakfast.

Fast Food

A fast diet is more harmful to the body than a benefit. If you can't wear this dress now, you can't wear it until this weekend. Changing food intake or diet to fruit or vegetables is not good for the body system. Your diet plan should be wisely chosen.

Regardless of the modification, you will need to choose a diet plan that includes all the essential nutrients and the type of food you need, as well as a certain amount. Your goal should be to keep your body working. If you expose yourself to food without calories, your body will have a hard time burning calories once you return to a normal diet.

Go out for Meal

One day in the week, eating out a lot of calorie food is not good for your health. Restaurant foods have higher calorie content than homemade foods, and you don't even know how many calories you need to consume. Research released by the Journal of Nutrition suggests women who eat homemade food lose weight.

Not those who eat once a week at the restaurant. You can limit your meal to at least once a month, and you'll be able to strike a balance between actually losing weight and achieving the health you need.

Learn How Japanese Maintain Their Weight

The main focus of Japanese dieting is to create health rather than maintain optimal weight. However, in the process of staying healthy, one will never eat food that causes obesity or overweight. Eating habits have no restrictions on your meal. Because there is no disease, the Japanese diet focuses on maintaining health, optimal weight, and enhanced immune function. The Japanese maintain their weight through practices that can be accepted by anyone. These methods have been around for centuries, and you might consider one of the following ways to stay healthy and maintain optimal immunity.

Avoid Milk

Milk combined with any meal provides excess calcium. The disadvantage of milk consumption is that the magnesium content of the food is insufficient. There is especially a lack of milk in the Japanese diet. Even if you eat milk, you can eat it alone without eating it with any other food or food. In addition, it must be noted that dairy products slow the rate of movement of the intestines and may ultimately fail to achieve the precise level of digestion required by the body, requiring additional tissue.

Optimize Food Temperature

People around the world often ignore food temperatures, but surprisingly, the Japanese tend to focus on food temperatures. They eat warm food in cold weather and cold meals in hot weather. In the summer, cold salads, celery, and other refrigerated foods are preferred, while in the winter, meat stews and different hot soups are preferred. High energy temperatures are critical to how the body reacts to our food. It is important to consider food temperature as part of a healthy eating habit.

Healthy Snack

Unlike Western food consisting of sugar and more sugar, Japanese snacks are healthier. They have replaced most of the biscuits and chips that are consumed in the West. They prefer sunflower seeds, pumpkin seeds, dried fruits, nuts, and seaweed snacks instead of cakes and biscuits. In addition to keeping you away from too much fat, these Japanese snacks also contain micronutrients, minerals, and vitamins.

Not Every Night Is a Sweet Night

The dessert night is very good because life is very important, so you should enjoy it. However, even for your child, you must place a dessert night at least once a week. This way, you will not consume more sugar than you need. If you want something to eat, please choose any fruit instead. This one Will keep your body away from excess fat-producing substances. Avoid using ice cream, biscuits, and sweet cakes to help you lose weight and help yourself.

Rice Combination

Take a combination of rice with stronger nutrition, such as purple rice, red rice, brown rice, or even black rice. Unpolished rice is also a good source of vitamin B. The whole rice should be eaten as a supplemental meal rather than the main way to avoid the constant fluctuations in sugar in the blood. When rice is consumed too much, it will affect the glycemic index due to sugar during digestion. Due to the low starch content, the rice combination is the preferred meal in the Japanese community. Rice blends also contain fewer calories.

Seafood

Seafood offers the best combination of healthy eating, and nutrition is especially good for the body and brain. The protein in the seafood keeps you happy for a long time and does not require snacks between meals. Asians practice eating fish every day, and an important part of the diet is not to refuse. Consider using all forms of seafood every day while staying healthy while maintaining a healthy weight. Starting with ordinary fish, you can resort to other types of seafood that can expand your cooking needs while achieving good health.

Small Plates and Chopsticks

Small plates and small bowls are needed to eat small amounts of food. There are also Asians, mainly Japanese who use chopsticks. This technique is a way to avoid shoveling food to your throat. In addition, the use of chopsticks will reduce the speed of eating, and in the end, you will reduce consumption and feel good. Although the use of chopsticks and small plates may require some discipline, they are especially needed for health.

3:1 Rationing

"The vegetables you want to eat are three times more than the meat."
This is an important recommendation for replacing healthy fat with a healthy meal that contains all the essential nutrients the body needs. Fill the table with vegetables instead of meat or other fat products. Include potatoes and other green vegetables in your diet to make sure you get the right combination. Flavored vegetables will also increase your appetite. Using spices on food will help your brain prefer vegetables, and eventually, you will need more vegetables than meat. In addition, fried vegetables should be avoided as much as possible.

Soup Plan

Soup is a densely nutritious food that fills you up immediately. The incredible thing about soup is that you don't need too much. All you need is the ability to prepare healthy soup, and you are ready. Bones and vegetables are the main combinations of Japanese soup. These meals contain enough vitamins and minerals to keep your body healthy for hours. The digestion is improved due to the high temperature of the soup. Therefore, if you are having trouble digesting, especially in the winter, you can also use warm soup.

Extreme Drink

Drinks should be kept to a minimum, usually cold drinks. In fact, health professionals have emphasized the importance of avoiding cold drinks or drinking water when eating hot food or just after eating hot food. Once you avoid cold drinks, it will promote better digestion of food. Digestive enzymes are not diluted. These proteins are critical to achieving optimal levels of absorption. Enzyme activity can be increased by eating hot or green tea, which is typical in the Japanese diet. Also, consider taking the liquid 30 minutes after a meal.

Conclusion

Have you tried different ways to get your body in good shape but found that most of them are not working? Are you willing to take an exciting method that can help you to not only attain your proper weight but also experience many benefits? If you answered yes to these questions, then this ultimate guide to intermittent fasting is you. With no fluff and straight to the point the book answers all the questions that you have been asking yourself about the 16:8 intermittent fasting. Intermittent fasting is the best way to go, and this book solves all the issues and answers various questions related to intermittent fasting.

Made in the USA
Columbia, SC
27 November 2019